P9-DEU-598

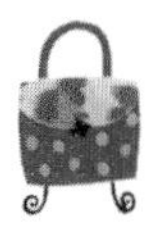

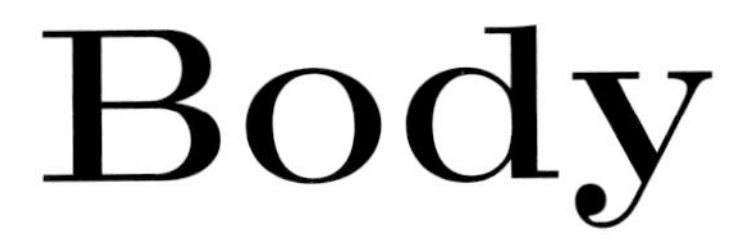

100 tips for a better body

Carol Morley & Liz Wilde

Time Warner Books

WARNER BOOKS
An AOL Time Warner Company

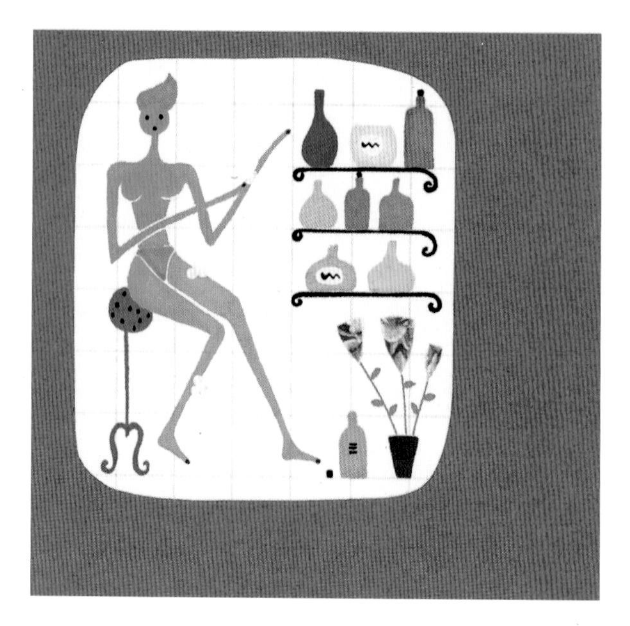

introduction

Looking for the body beautiful? From smooth, toned legs to tight abs, from a tranquil mind to a pampered body, these professional tips will get you in shape. Feel healthy from the inside out; treat your body with the respect it deserves, and you will be rewarded with a supple figure and tons of energy. Love your natural body shape—and make the very most of what you've got!

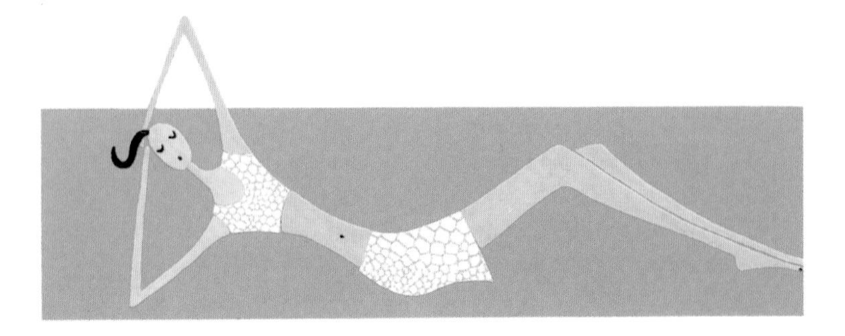

contents

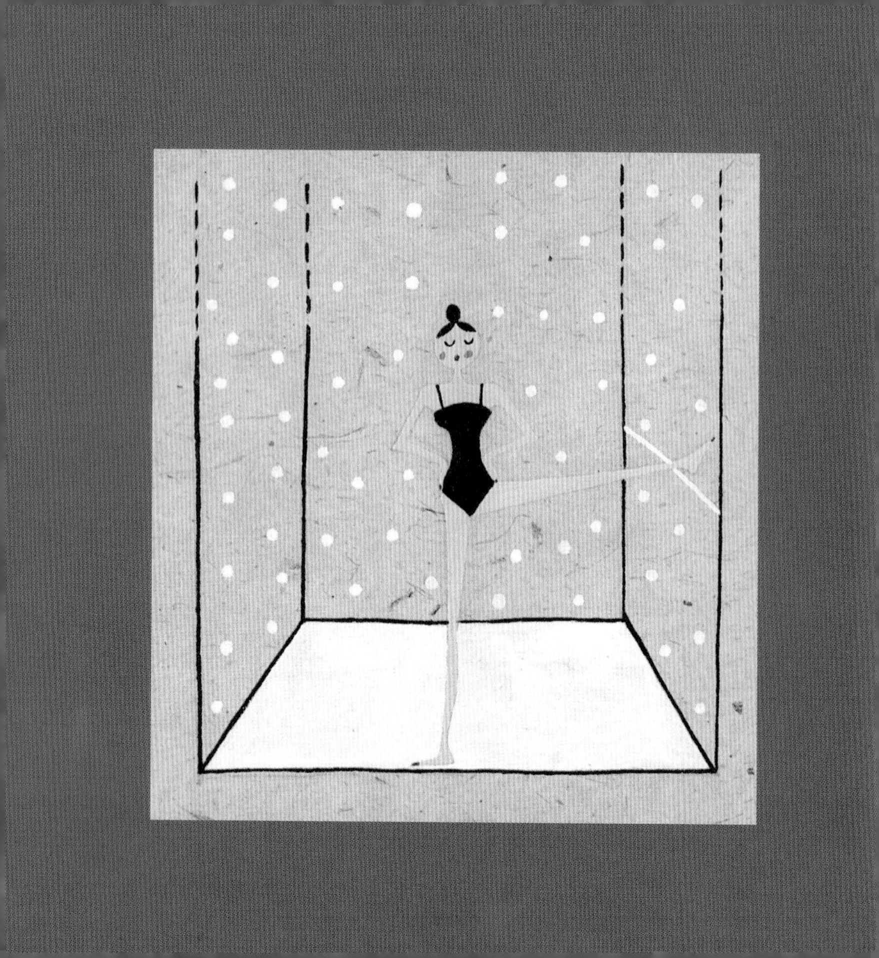

chapter 1

Healthy body

1 **Studies show that too many of us don't get enough sleep.** If you suffer from headaches, mood swings, irritability, memory loss, or weepiness, chances are you're sleep deprived. If you find you are missing out on sleep during the week, try and catch up over the weekend. Add a sleep inducing essential oil (lavender, neroli, camomile, or mandarin) to your evening bath to help you fall asleep if you're having trouble relaxing.

2 **To ensure a peaceful night's sleep,** avoid alcohol, nicotine, and caffeine for at least four hours before you slip between the sheets.

3 **If you regularly go to bed with your mind racing,** try a little meditation before you lay your head down. Dim the lights and focus on a point about three feet away. Inhale deeply through your nose and then exhale through your mouth. If your mind starts to wander, bring it back by concentrating on your breathing.

4 **Follow your cat's example and start the day with a slow stretch.** Then take a deep breath in through your nose right down to your diaphragm, hold for a few seconds, and push it slowly out. Repeat four times and you'll feel clearheaded and ready for the day.

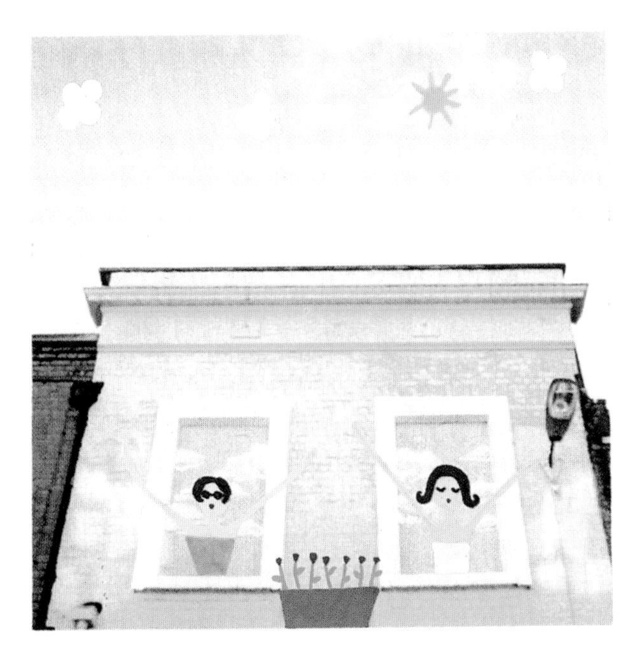

5 **No amount of dieting or exercise will change your basic body shape.** But the right exercise can improve fitness and muscle tone and help you make the most of your natural body shape. There are thousands of different bodies out there, but everyone conforms to these three basic types:

Endomorphs (think Drew Barrymore) have the roundest body types with plenty of curves. Women with this body type tend to store body fat more easily than others and have hips wider than their shoulders. The best exercise for this type concentrates on cardiovascular work to burn fat and streamline curves.

Mesomorphs (think Madonna) have fairly large bones and their shoulders are a little wider than their hips. This is the squarest body type and tends to be naturally muscular. If you have this body type, keep in mind that weight training will cause you to build up bulky muscle quickly.

Ectomorphs (think supermodel) are the traditional beanpoles—small boned and skinny. Their shoulders and hips are the same size and it's harder for them to build muscle. Ectomorphs need to improve their muscle definition through strength training, not by hours burning fat on a treadmill.

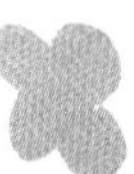

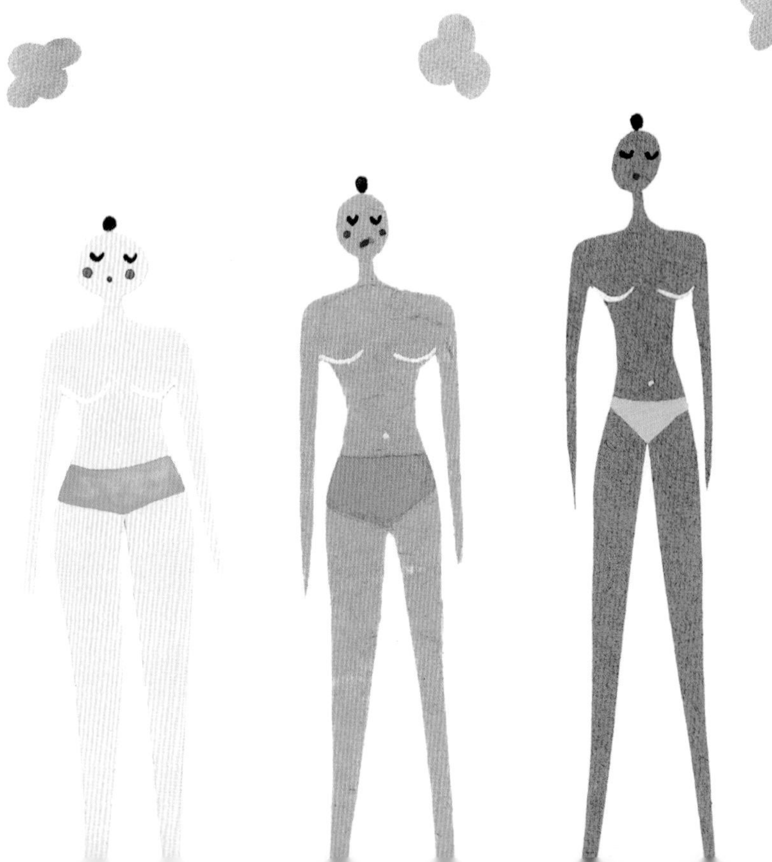

6 **Standing up straight will make you look slimmer.** Forget the old finishing school trick of balancing a book on your head. All you need to do is imagine a string is pulling you up from the center of your head. Relax the rest of your body and look in the mirror. Your bottom will be tucked under and your tummy will be tucked in. Good posture also promotes better breathing by allowing your diaphragm to fully extend, and walking tall gives you confidence.

7 **Why wait for someone else to give you a massage?** When you're feeling tense, lie on your side and massage the side and back of your neck in slow circles. Move down to your shoulders and as far as you can reach on your back. Repeat on the other side.

8 **When you feel worn out,** try pinching the point between your thumb and forefinger for two minutes. This acupressure area is said to release instant energy.

9 **The adrenaline rush set off by a stressful situation** equals enough energy to power a mile run, and it diverts energy away from where you need it. No surprise that after a stressful day you feel worn out. Next time you feel the tension rising, take a walk, count to 10, or breathe deeply—anything to calm you down.

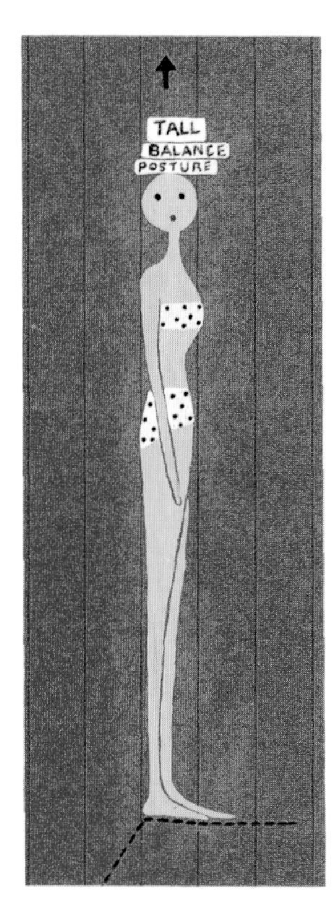
TALL
BALANCE
POSTURE

10 **While you can live without food for a while,** only a few days without water are enough to kill you. Your body is made up of around 65 percent water and this level needs constant replenishing or you'll feel tired. Exposure to central heating and air conditioning accelerates water loss from the body, and a diet high in salt, sugar, or food additives may also contribute to dehydration. The recommended daily water intake is eight to ten 8oz glasses—you will need even more if you exercise. Check your urine—pale yellow means you are getting enough; any darker means you're not.

11 **Ditch that coffee.** Instead, start the day with a cup of hot water containing the juice of half a lemon to refresh your body and cleanse your liver. Hot water with lemon is especially beneficial after an alcohol-fueled night out (or in).

Healthy body

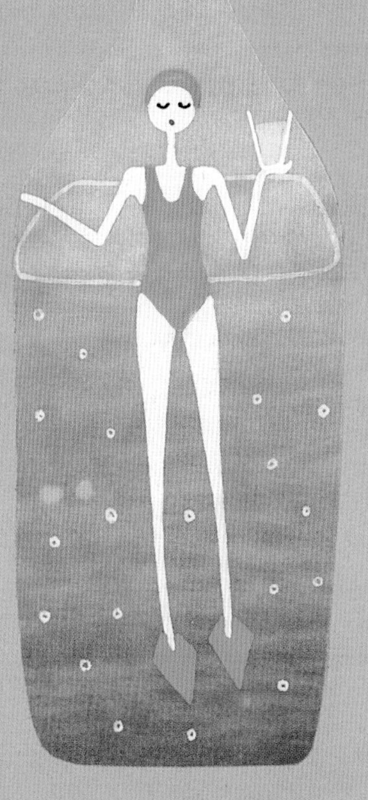

12 **Healthy eating means feeling great.** Here's what you should aim to include in your diet each day:

- *One serving of protein (fish, meat, cheese, eggs, soya, nuts, seeds).*
- *Five servings of vegetables and fruit (organic is best).*
- *One serving (at least) of carbohydrates (rice, potatoes, beans, lentils, pasta, up to four slices of bread).*
- *Between eight and ten 8oz glasses of pure, still water.*
- *One teaspoon (at least) of extra virgin olive oil.*

13 **Ever wondered why experts** go on and on about eating more fruit and vegetables? Well, not only are these foods rich in vitamins, minerals, and fiber, they also contain antioxidants, which help prevent cancer and heart disease, and flavonoids, which fight everyday infections and viruses.

14 **Eat some yogurt with live cultures every day** as it helps improve digestion and ease common conditions such as irritable bowel syndrome.

15 **When choosing rice, pasta, and bread,** look for the words "unrefined" and "whole" on the label. These contain more fiber and vitamin B than the standard products, so they will give your body better slow-release energy.

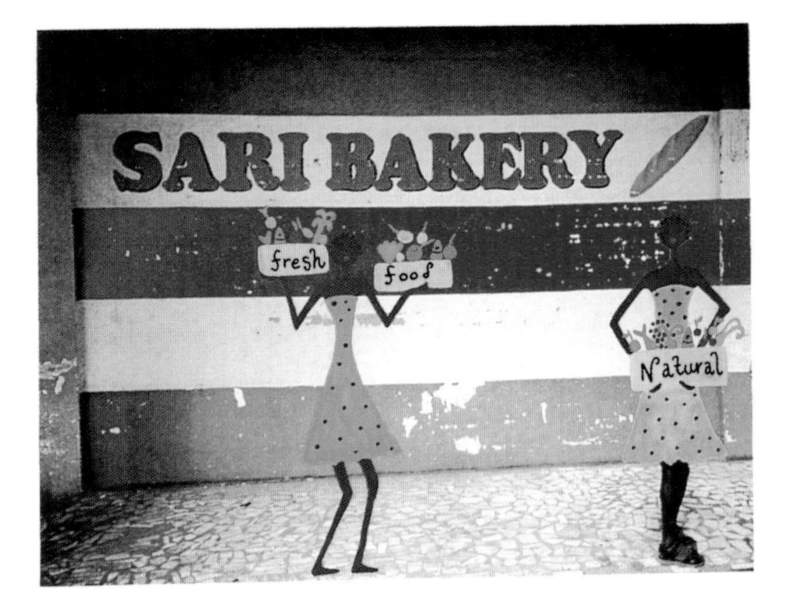
SARI BAKERY
fresh
food
Natural

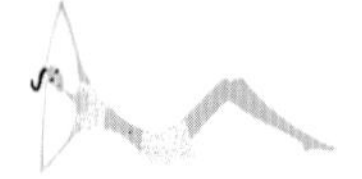

16 **Getting fit doesn't have to mean sweating it out at the gym.** When the weather's warm (and even when it's not), outdoor sports are a great way to improve your fitness and your body.

Rowing is excellent for tightening the stomach and toning your upper body—concentrate on using your buttocks as you pull up to work your lower body, too.

Basketball makes a speedy cardio-vascular workout that burns fat and builds up muscle in your legs.

Swimming the front crawl will give you an overall toner, and the breast stroke is great for toning thighs and shoulders.

Soccer gives your whole body a total work out. Ninety minutes spent running around will burn fat and tone your legs fast.

Golf is a more gentle workout for body and mind. Swinging the club and hitting the ball tones up arms and shoulders and walking briskly around the course boosts the heart rate.

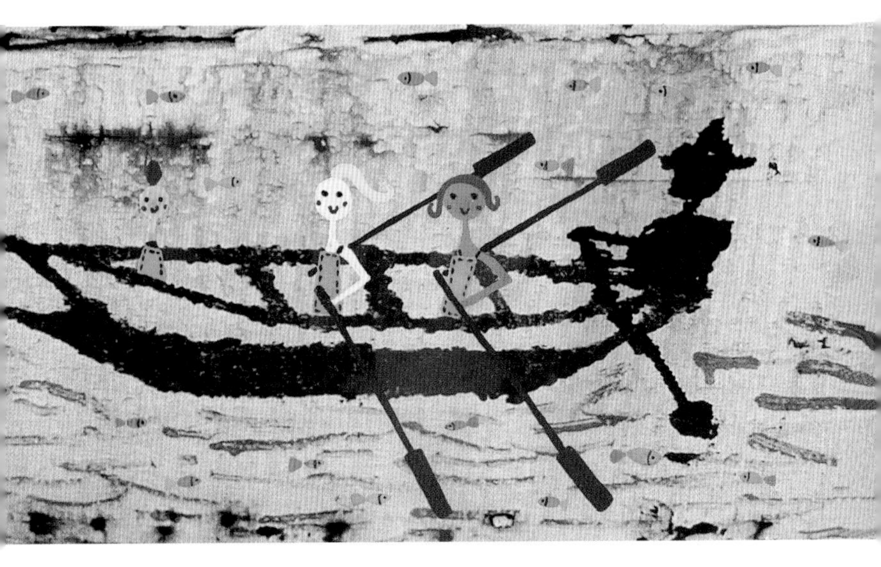

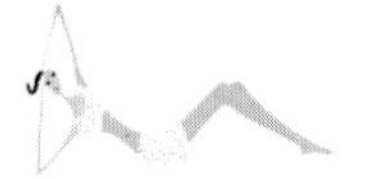

17 **Why exercise? Here are ten good reasons:**

1. Boosts your immune system.
2. Helps maintain your ideal body weight.
3. Relieves stress.
4. Lifts depression.
5. Relieves PMS.
6. Encourages sound sleep.
7. Improves skin.
8. Promotes healthy hair.
9. Increases your energy.
10. Tones your muscles.

18 **Dancing is a great exercise as it burns calories, improves your mood**—and doesn't feel like exercise at all. Next time you're at the disco, instead of sticking wallflower-like to the bar, get out on the dance floor and shake your bootie. A night of jiggling around is the equivalent of the toughest aerobics class. Too shy to shimmy in front of others? Then wait until the house is empty, put on your favorite album and dance around your room. It'll make you feel better instantly, and regular dancing around at home will help tone and tighten any flabby parts of your body. You never know, you may get so good you'll be taking over the dance floor in no time!

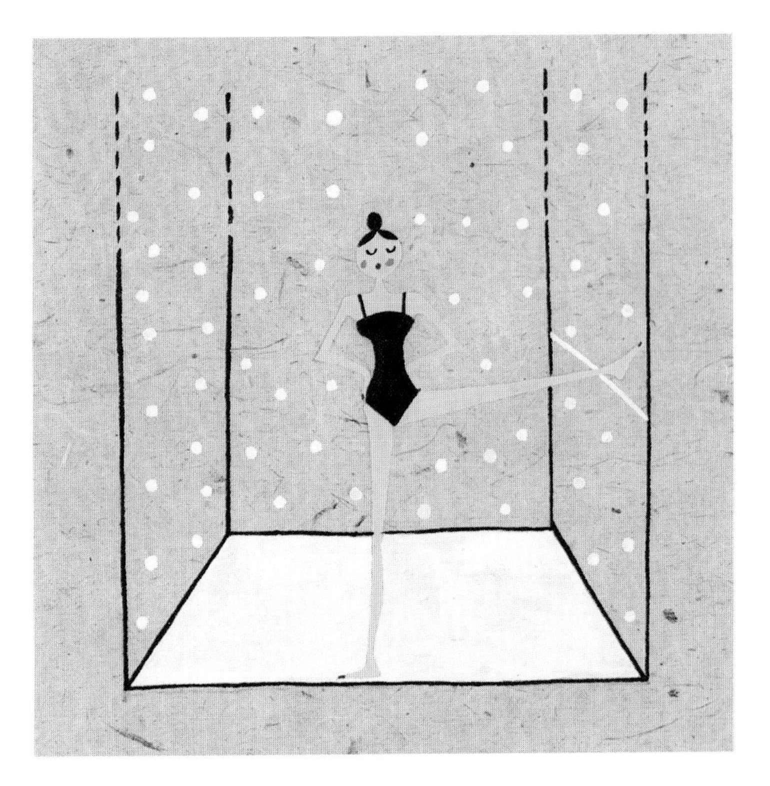

19 **There's no such thing as a healthy tan.** But if you're determined to be outside, there are a few simple rules you must follow if you want to keep your skin wrinkle-free and avoid potentially fatal skin cancer. And remember, sunlight is responsible for at least 80 percent of ageing.

- *Cover up. Put on a hat and slip on a shirt.*
- *Always use a sunscreen that protects against ageing UVA rays and has an SPF 15 or more to protect from burning UVB rays.*
- *Don't skimp on your sunscreen. If used correctly, an average person should only get four or five applications out of a 4-ounce bottle.*
- *Buy a new sunscreen every year as bacteria will grow inside the bottle during the winter (especially if you store the bottle in a warm bathroom) and kill off its power against the sun.*

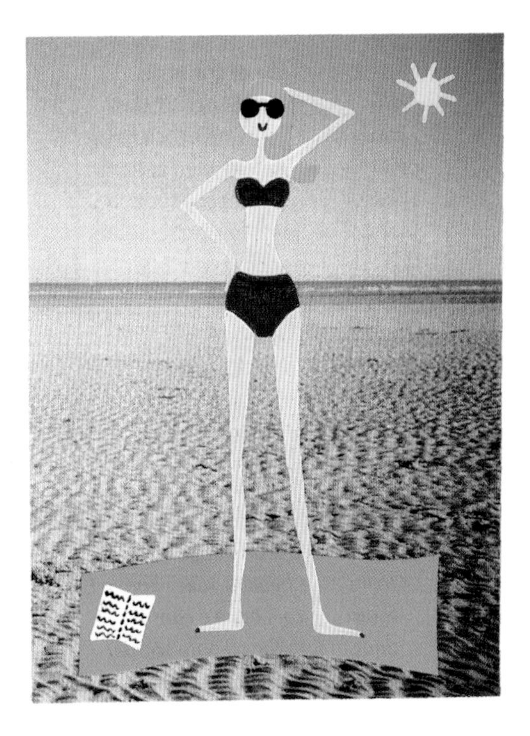

20 **Every case of sunburn increases your chance of skin cancer,** but it's a rare beach babe who hasn't been burned at least once. If your skin needs soothing, try one of the following remedies.

- *Mix half a cup of milk with a pinch of baking soda.*
- *Mix 2 tablespoons of vinegar and a cup of water.*
- *Smooth on calamine lotion.*
- *Add a few drops of camomile oil to your bath water.*
- *Lavender oil will help heal blistered skin; use undiluted.*
- *To improve healing, take vitamin E tablets, or split open a capsule and smooth the oil onto scarred or damaged skin.*

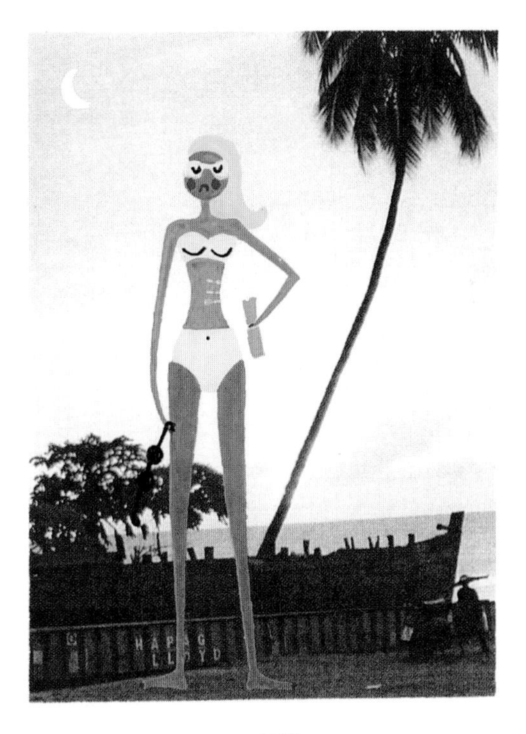

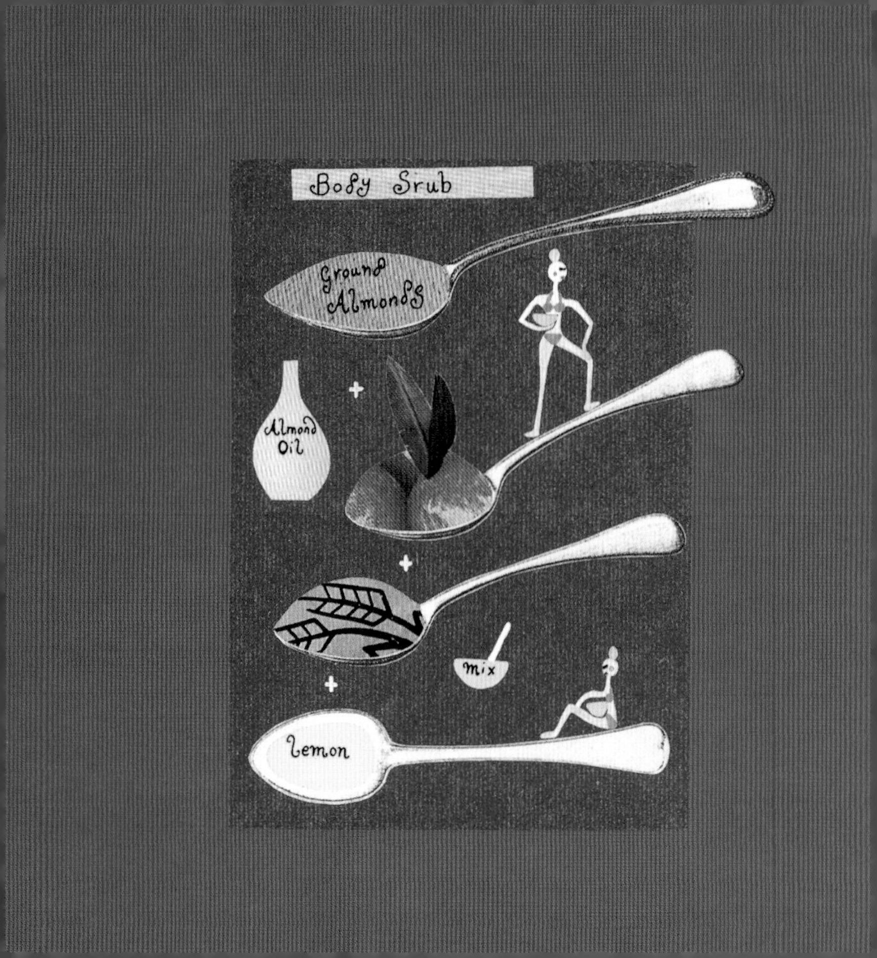

Body Srub
Ground Almonds
Almond Oil
+
+
+
mix
lemon

chapter 2

Smooth body

The people in some countries think body hair is attractive. Unfortunately, we don't live in one of them, so most of us fight a constant battle to banish our unwanted hair. But don't forget, you have a choice...

21 **Shaving is quick, cheap, and painless** (unless you cut yourself). You'll have to do it daily if you want supersmooth skin and change the blade every six shaves. The best place to shave is in the bath or shower. Wait a few minutes for your hair to soften in the water before you start. Using shaving cream or gel will leave your skin softer than soap.

22 **Consider investing in an epilator only if you have a high pain threshold.** These handheld electronic devices have rotating metal blades that trap the hairs and pull them out at the root. Products that promise to numb the skin may make it a little less painful, but this method is never going to be a pleasure.

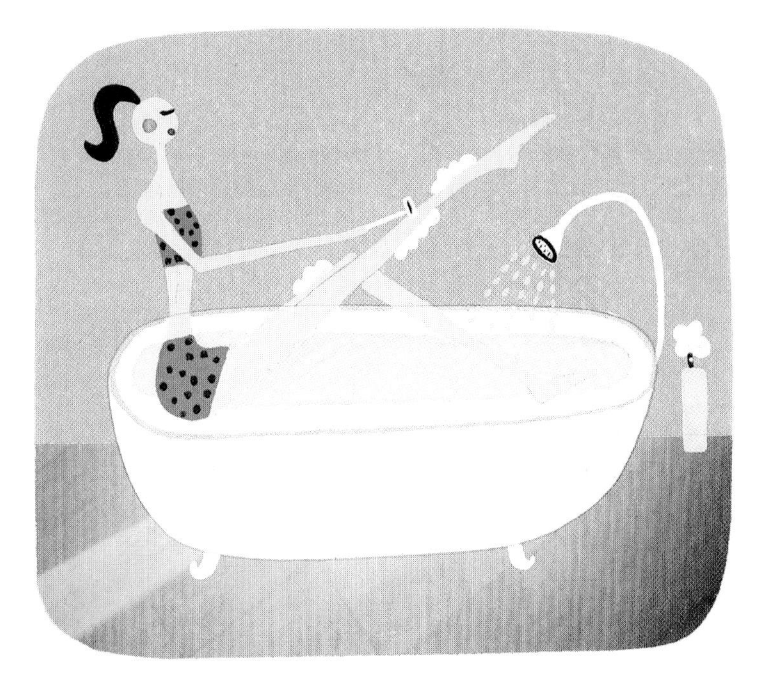

23 **Hair-removing creams give long-lasting results with no stubble,** but they take time (about 10 to 15 minutes) and can be messy and smelly—no matter what the "perfumed" product promises. Expect results to last about two weeks, and you'll need to avoid sunscreens, body lotions, and self tanners for a few hours after defuzzing to avoid irritation. Depilatory virgins should do a patch test first to make sure their skin's not sensitive.

24 **Not so long ago, the only permanent hair removal was electrolysis.** Now we have a method of hair removal that uses sound waves, which promises to be far less painful because no needles stick into the skin. Tweezers are passed over the surface, and a current is sent directly down the hair follicle to destroy the root. And after a short course of treatments, your hair growth will gradually become weaker and slower until it stops.

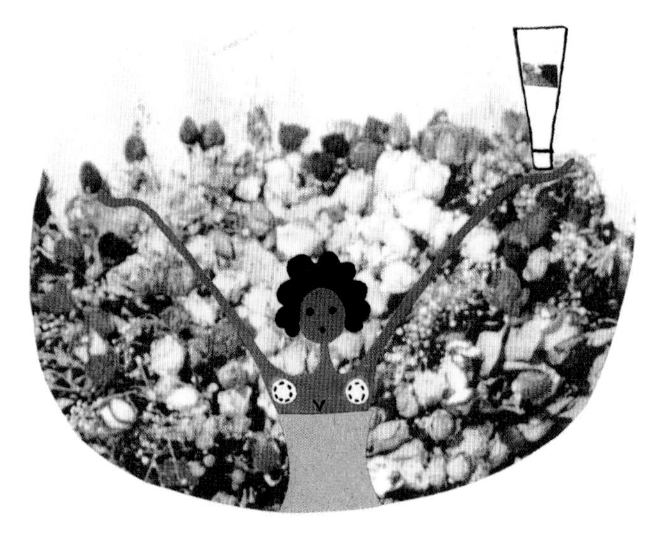

25 **Waxing gives the longest-lasting results of all temporary forms of hair removal.** Fine hairs reappear after about two weeks, and thicker ones after about four. Hair also becomes finer the longer you wax, which is just as well since it has to be half an inch long before you can rewax. But beware—waxing is painful. Avoid too much agony by holding your skin taut before pulling the wax away, and try breathing in and then out as you pull—it helps takes the sting away. Don't wax immediately before you go on vacation as you should keep newly waxed skin away from the sun and sunscreen for a couple of days.

26 **Sugaring is an old Eastern technique similar to waxing** that promises to be less painful because the sugary paste sticks to your hair rather than your skin. Still, don't expect a picnic.

Homemade sugaring recipe:
1. Melt 1 pound of sugar together with the juice of two lemons. Simmer for 10 minutes and add 1½ teaspoons of glycerine.
2. Apply the warm mixture in thin downward strips.
3. Press a piece of cloth over the top and pull back toward you.

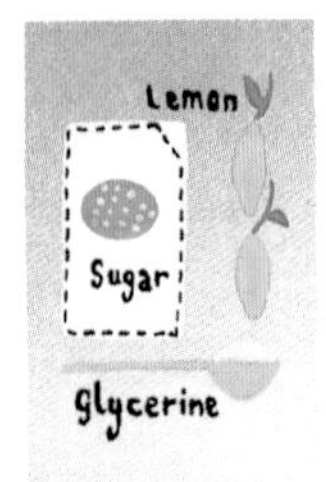

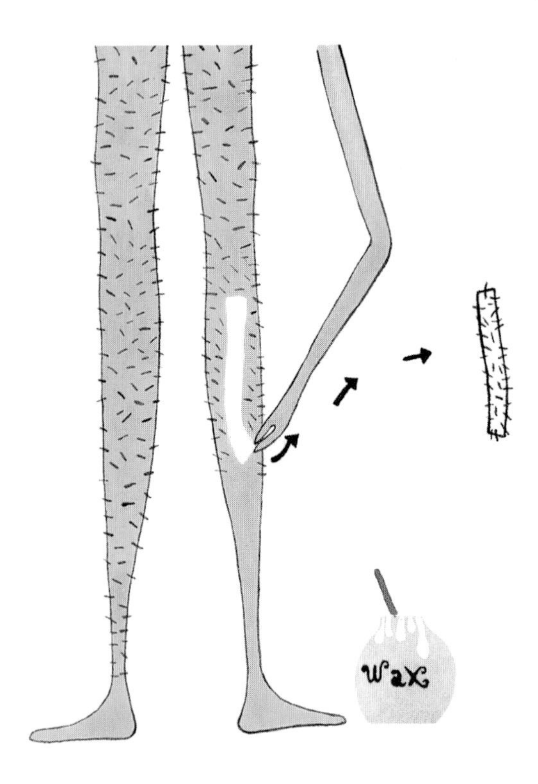
wax

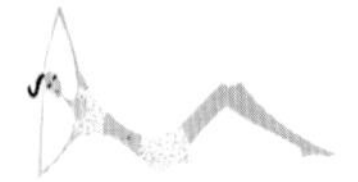

27 **Beauty therapists swear by body brushing,** but expect a little discomfort when you start. The idea is to brush your skin before showering with a soft-bristle body brush using long, sweeping movements. This not only removes dead skin cells in one swoop but stimulates lymphatic drainage, which encourages elimination of up to a third of your body's waste. The rule is to start at the farthest point from your heart (ie. feet or hands) and work inward. Start with gentle brushing, and as you become used to the tingling, increase the pressure. We promise it becomes almost pleasurable. Keep your brush clean (think of all those nasty dead skin cells trapped in the bristles) and if you really can't bear a brush, use a loofah or towel instead.

28 **Ingrown hairs look like sore, red spots.** The tip of the hair gets embedded in dead skin cells and starts growing under the skin. Avoid ingrown hairs by gently exfoliating with a loofah or massage mitt to keep pores free from dead skin buildup. Don't apply body lotion immediately after waxing. It may feel soothing, but the cream will only block pores and trap hairs.

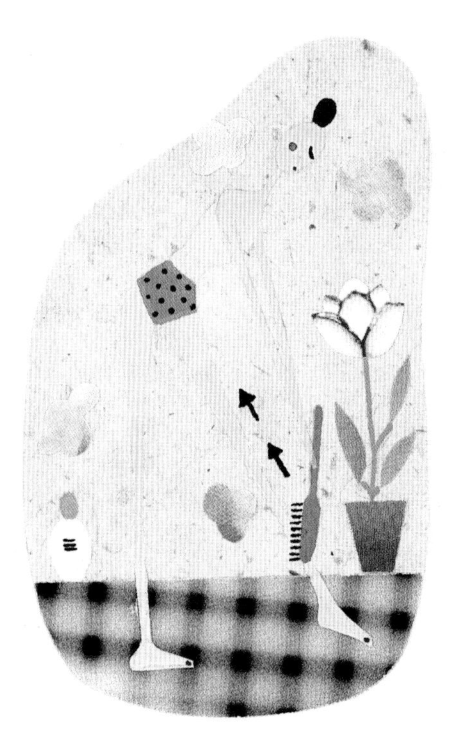

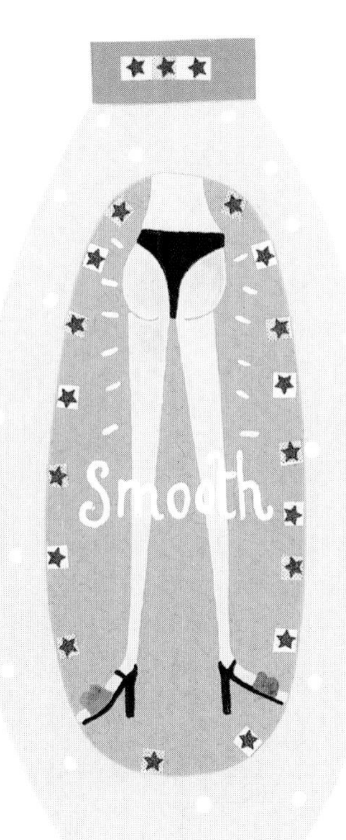
Smooth

29 **Don't believe the hype.** A cream can smooth your skin but it can't firm up your body. Only exercise will do that.

30 **Body creams now promise the same miracles as face creams.** But a far cheaper alternative is wheat-germ oil, which has a similar structure to sebum (the skin's natural oil) and also contains conditioning vitamins A, B, C, and E.

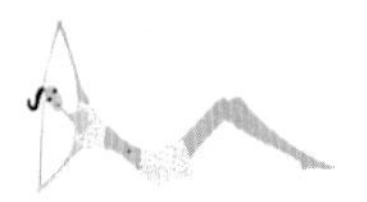

31 Skin renews itself every 28 days, but the process slows down as we grow older. Get into the habit of exfoliating your skin once a week and it'll feel smoother, softer, and look more radiant. Use a loofah, massage mitt, or body scrub and work on damp skin (a shower's the best scrub zone) using gentle, circular movements. Pay special attention to areas that are always dry (think knees, elbows, and feet) and follow with a generous application of moisturizer.

32 For a luxurious home scrub, whip up this recipe:

- *1 tablespoon of dried, finely ground orange peel*
- *1 tablespoon of dried, finely ground lemon peel*
- *2 tablespoons of ground almonds*
- *4 tablespoons of oatmeal*
- *Enough almond oil to make a paste*
- *2 drops of essential oil, to perfume*

Mix all the ingredients together and rub onto damp skin in gentle, circular motions. Rinse with clean water.

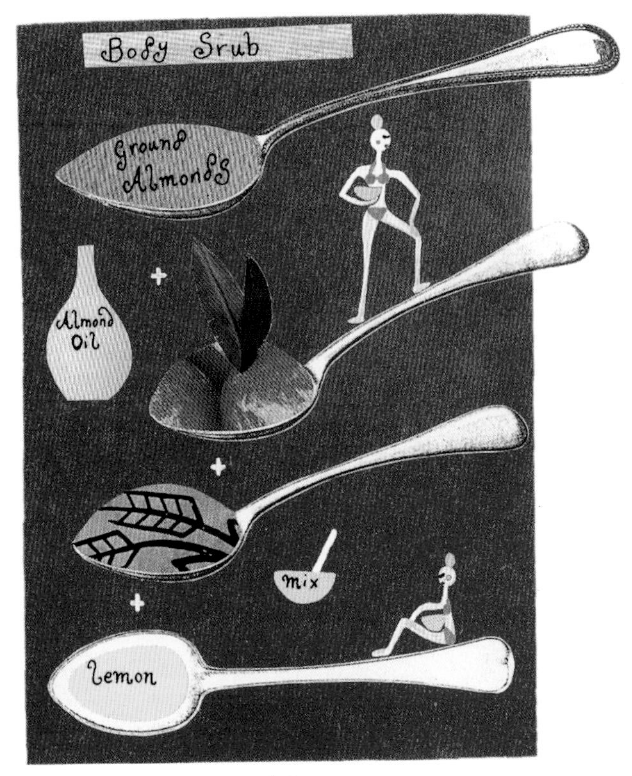
Body Srub
Ground Almonds
Almond Oil
mix
Lemon

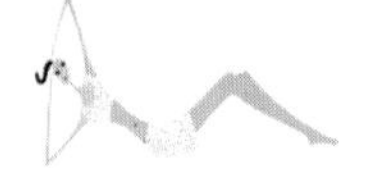

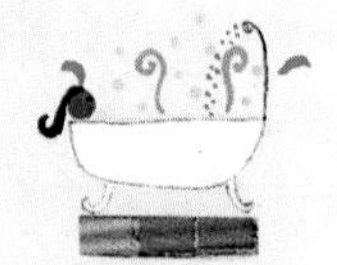

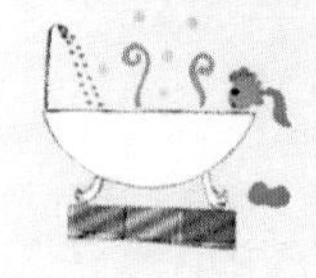

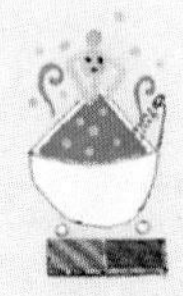

33 The bathtub is more than just a place to get your body clean. It can deeply relax you, soothe sore muscles, relieve aches and pains, flush away toxins, and dislodge dirt, sweat, and dead skin cells too. It all comes down to what you put in the water.

- *Epsom salts will relax tired muscles and joints.*
- *Sea salt will give you a deep down cleanse as you scrub.*
- *Cider or wine vinegar soothes dry skin.*
- *Powdered skimmed milk moisturizes.*
- *A few drops of aromatherapy oil added after the water has run will soothe your skin.*
- *A drop of your favorite perfume will make the water (and you) smell sweeter.*

34 Don't make your bath water too warm—the recommended temperature is around 80 degrees—or your pulse will race and you'll feel drained after your dunking. Very hot water will also remove too much of your skin's natural sebum, which helps hold moisture. And don't wallow too long—30 minutes tops. You want to come out with soft, not shriveled, skin.

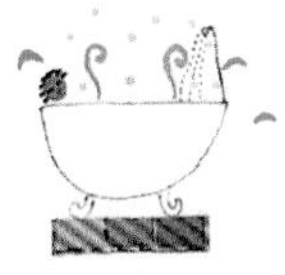

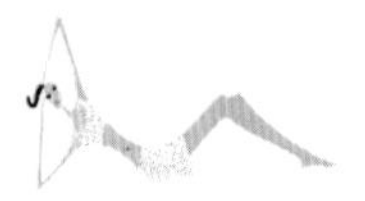

35 **Any cleanser you use that lathers up contains a detergent.** So whether you choose soap or shower gel, make sure you moisturize afterward. For extra mildness, buy translucent glycerine soaps: They are low-lather and rinse away quickly. Sensitive skin will love honey and milk products, and dry skin will soak up any product labeled "moisturizing." Oh, and try putting rubber bands around bottle tops to improve your slippery grip in the shower.

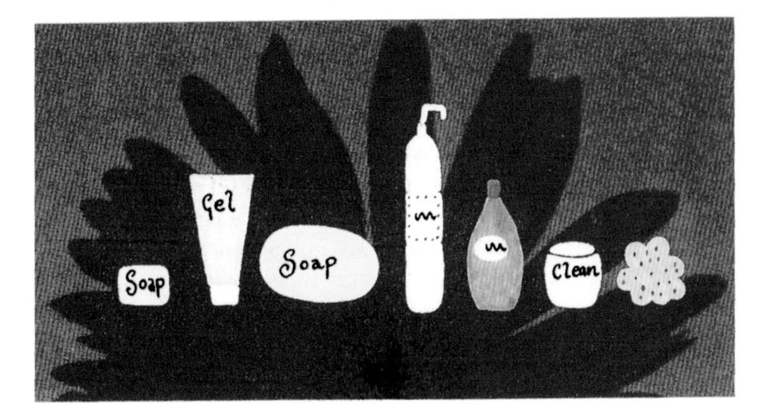
Gel
Soap
Soap
Clean

36 **After you've had a bath is the best time to moisturize.** Smooth on a hydrator while your skin's still damp and it'll lock in extra moisture. And if you've got a few extra minutes to spare, give your problem areas a quick massage to improve circulation and encourage toxins to leave town. Use your fingertips and palms, working in firm, deep-kneading movements all over those knotted muscles.

37 **Manufacturers would have us believe that we need a different cream for every part of the body.** Not all skin is created equal (some areas are thicker than others), which is why creams sink in quickly on certain parts of you (elbows, knees, and ankles drink up moisture immediately). As a rule, you can use the same body lotion on every part of you—but don't use a body product on your face, which is extra sensitive.

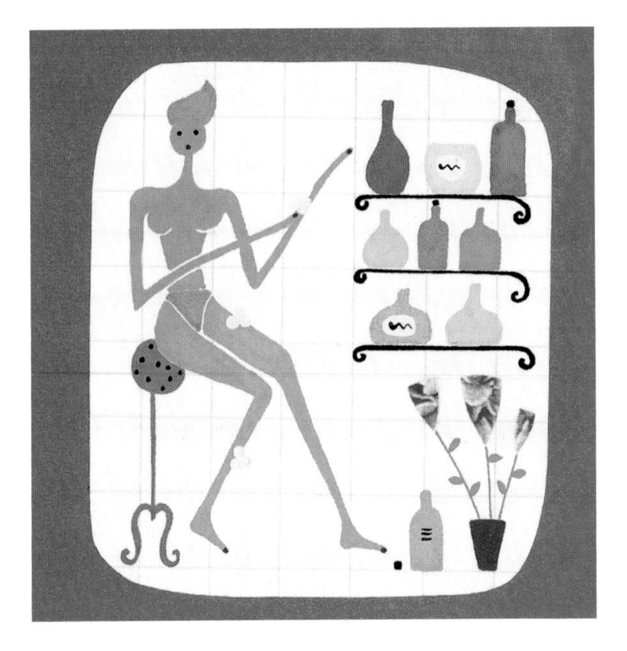

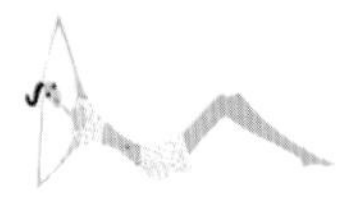

38 **Honey is a natural healer** found in many moisturizers. Because they attract and hold in moisture, honey-based products are ideal for the very dry.

39 **Make your own body scrub** with a handful of sea salt or sugar mixed with your usual cleanser. If your skin is very dry mix the salt or sugar with honey or vegetable oil for a moisturizing scrub.

40 **Even the driest, toughest skin will respond to a little looking after,** but don't expect results overnight. Concentrate on building up a routine—your skin will thank you for it!

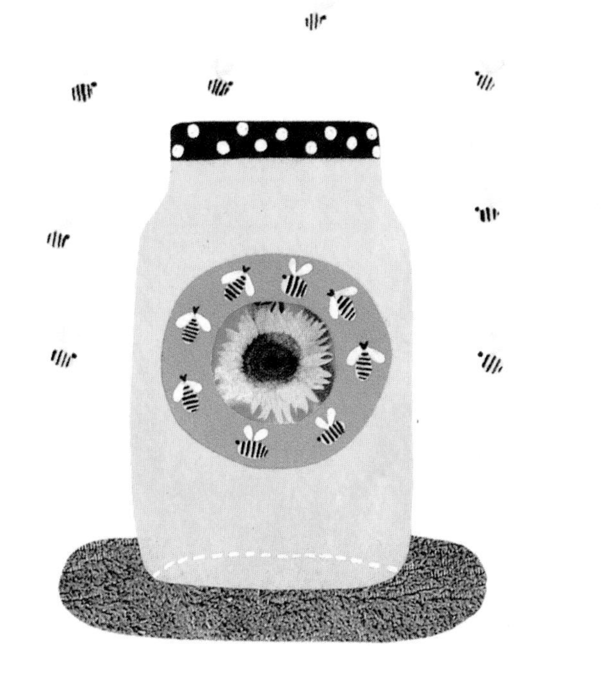

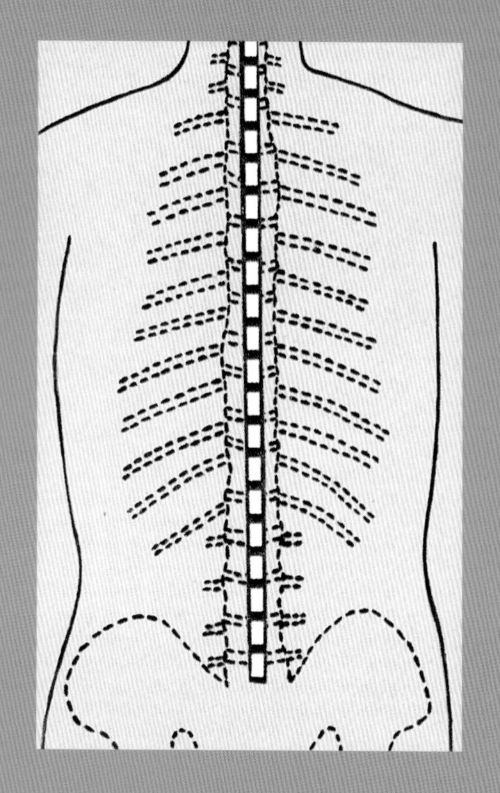

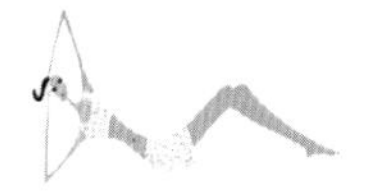

chapter 3

Upper body

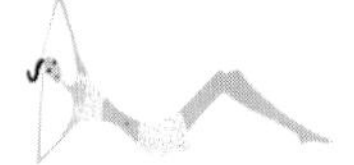

41 **Your neck will give your age away.** Fewer fat cells and oil producing glands in this area make for skin that's extra thin and dry. Remember your neck in your skin-care regimen and always smooth creams upward—why give gravity any help?

42 **The skin between your neck and breasts** (known as your décolletage) is extra thin and usually the first part of you to burn. Protect it with a high SPF sunscreen and moisturize daily. Sleeping on your side will also leave you creased come morning, so when you slather on your nighttime moisturizer, extend it down to your chest. You'll wake up looking far less folded.

43 **It's easy to ignore your back,** but when out of sight means out of mind, you could be in for a nasty shock. Pimples love all those extra oil glands behind you, so if you're suffering, use a tea tree oil wash on your break-out area. And if your back's very bad, a trip to the dermatologist will sort it out.

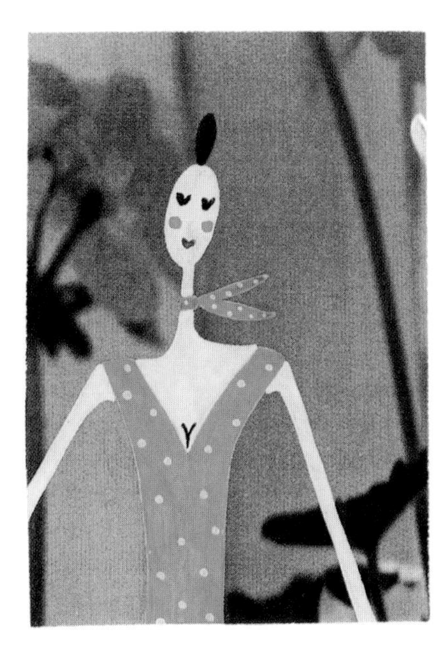

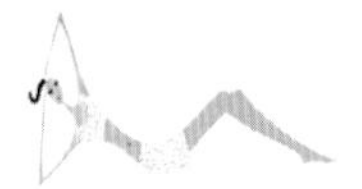

44 Perfect posture will transform your upper body. No more rounded shoulders and droopy bustline. Try this exercise:

1. Stand with your heels a couple of inches from a wall with your feet hip-width apart.

2. Slowly press your body backwards, keeping your toes on the floor. Just your hair, shoulder blades, and bottom should touch the wall.

3. If your shoulders are way out, you need to do a little corrective work. Imagine that someone's pulling you up by a piece of string attached to the top of your head. When you feel an inch taller, relax your shoulders. You probably look like you just gained a whole cup size, too.

45 Forget expensive toning creams. Splash your breasts with cold water for the cheapest bust tightener in town.

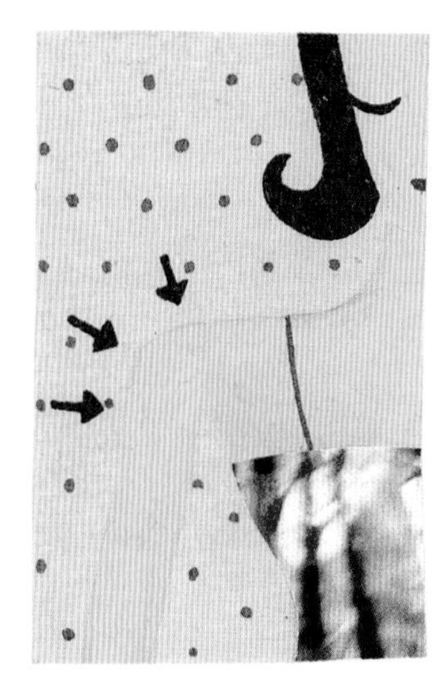

46 When sweat pumps out of your pores, it's completely odorless. It's only when bacteria gets involved that the smell starts, and that takes about six hours. You have two underarm options: antiperspirants, which contain chemicals to reduce sweating and bacteria, or deodorants, which mask odor. Some people prefer not to tamper with their bodies' natural cooling system, while others hate to get wet (smell or no smell). The choice is yours.

47 The natural way to combat sweat is with a crystal deodorant. Made from mineral salts, these work by inhibiting bacterial growth, and no bacteria means no odor. Just wet the end of the crystal before using. Each stick will last far longer than your average antiperspirant.

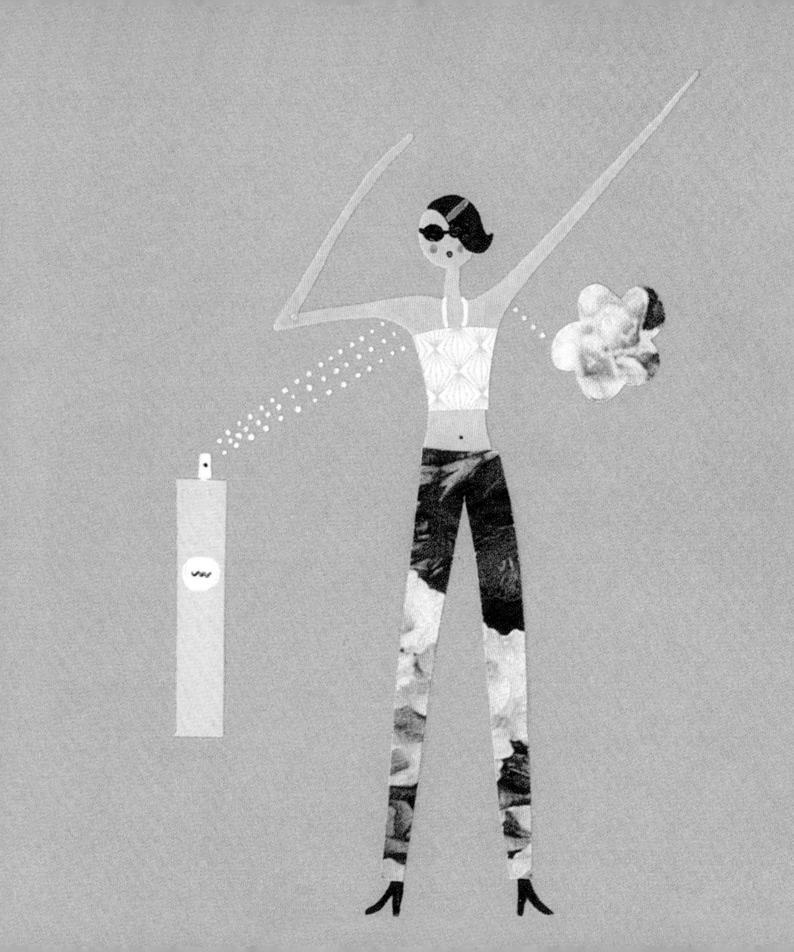

48 Exercise will firm your breasts, but don't expect miracles. Your breasts are made of milk glands surrounded by fatty tissue. What you're actually exercising is the supporting muscles that keep them lifted.

1. Stand facing a wall with arms out and palms flat against it at shoulder height. Breathe in and lean your body as close to the wall as you can, then breathe out and push back to the starting position. Aim for 15.

2. Holding small hand weights, stand tall with your arms straight out to the sides at shoulder level. Slowly rotate your arms forward, aiming for 20 small circles, then repeat going backward for 20.

3. Stand tall with your hands clasped together at chest height. Now push your palms together hard for a count of five and release, repeating 10 times.

49 Rough bumpy skin appears on the upper arms due to poor circulation. Make it disappear by giving it a good scrub in the shower. Use a massage mitt in firm circular movements, then smooth on a moisturizer.

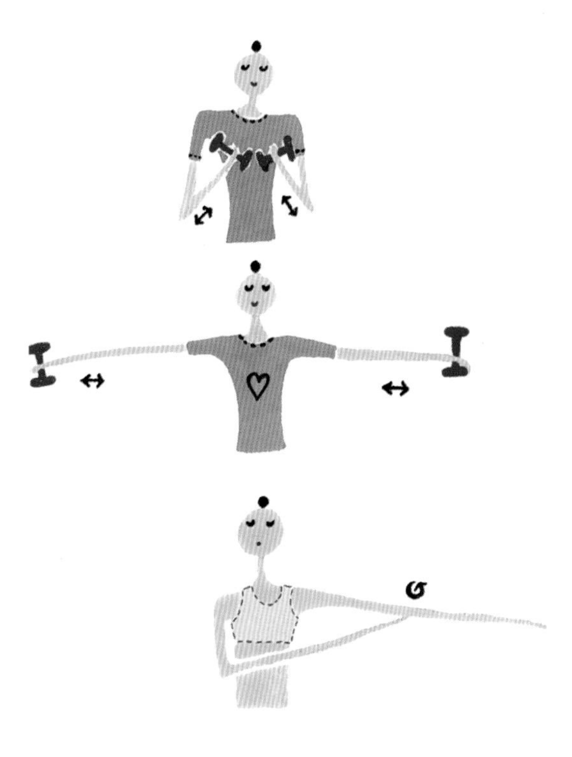

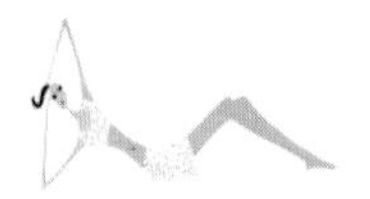

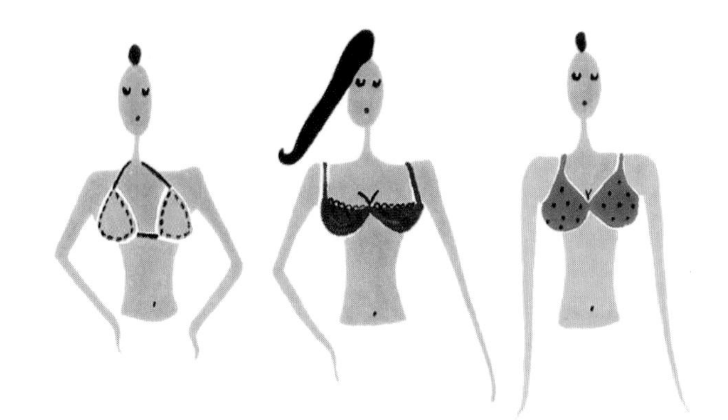

50 The right bra can create a cleavage, minimize, support, or add inches.

- *Halter-neck styles stop you from bouncing in backless dresses.*
- *Underwire push-up bras make the most of very little.*
- *Seemless cups look invisible under sheer fabrics.*
- *Strapless styles keep you uplifted in the skimpiest of outfits.*
- *Sports bras are a must during exercise for preventing droop.*
- *Bandeau bras can flatten too-full figures.*

Remember to wash a new bra before wearing it for the first time—this will help it conform to your body shape.

51 **Just because you can get a bra on doesn't mean it fits.** If you want your breasts to look their best, you need a well-fitting bra. There are lots of reasons why your bra size might change (losing or gaining weight, having a baby, etc). If you're too shy to be measured by a stranger, here's how to do it yourself. Wrap a tape measure just under your breasts around your back—making sure the tape's in a straight line and feels comfortable. This measurement in inches is your bra size. Next, measure around the fullest part of your bust. The difference between the two measurements is your cup size. If it is the same as your bra size you need an A cup, a 1-inch difference is a B cup, a 2-inch difference is a C cup, and so on. For the best fit, visit the underwear department in your local store, where you can get expert advice. The only way to ensure a perfect fit is trial and error and there are plenty of styles to try.

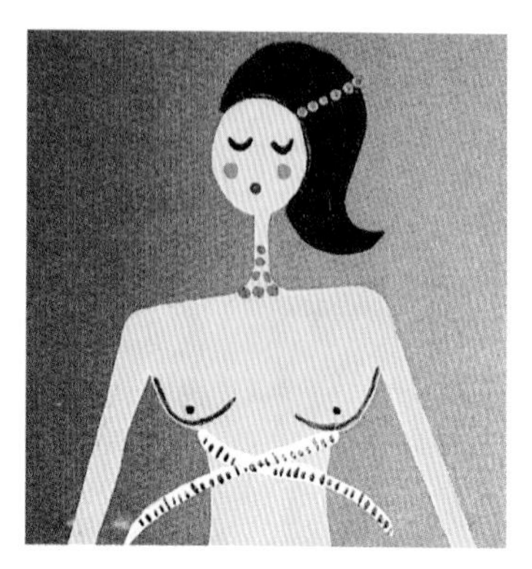

52 **Every woman should examine her breasts once a month during the week after the end of her period.** Try and make it part of your regular routine, so that you notice any changes or anything unusual. Why? Because early detection is the best weapon against breast cancer.

1. Raise your right arm above your head, and feel the whole breast and armpit using the fingers of your left hand. Work in small circles with firm pressure, feeling for any lumps or hardened areas. Repeat on the other side.

2. Lie on your back with a pillow under your right shoulder. With your right hand under your head, check your right breast as you did before, and then swap to the other side and check that in the same way.

If you do find a lump or anything suspicious, don't panic. It doesn't mean you've got breast cancer—but you should make a doctor's appointment.

53 **It's perfectly normal for one of your breasts to be larger than the other.** Women who've had breast enlargement surgery have even been known to complain that their perfectly matched breasts didn't look natural, so be proud of your differences!

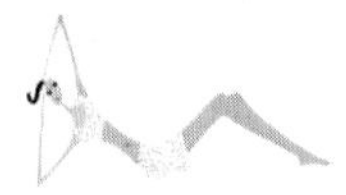

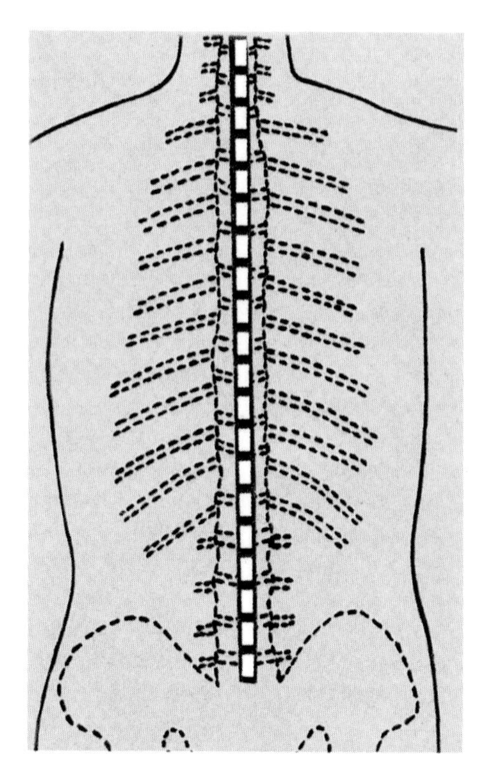

54 **About 80 percent of back problems are caused by weak muscles.** Pilates is an exercise technique that strengthens and lengthens the muscles through a series of slow, controlled movements centering on the abdomen. It does wonders for a weak back (and a saggy stomach), because before every movement, you need to tuck in your pelvis and hold it steady—which means serious middle body strengthening.

55 **Crunching away everyday and still no washboard stomach?** It may be that you're not doing it right. You need to keep the movements slow and steady, counting three seconds up and then three down (yes, that slow). Breathe out as you come up, and really concentrate on the muscles you're working. They'll reward you by becoming strong, lean fibers that will eventually make your sit-ups a breeze (and more important, your stomach fit for baring).

56 **Sit-ups don't actually get rid of fat.** What they will do is strengthen the muscles lying over your stomach to hold it tightly in place. The layer of fat over the top needs a combination of healthy eating and heart-racing exercise to disappear.

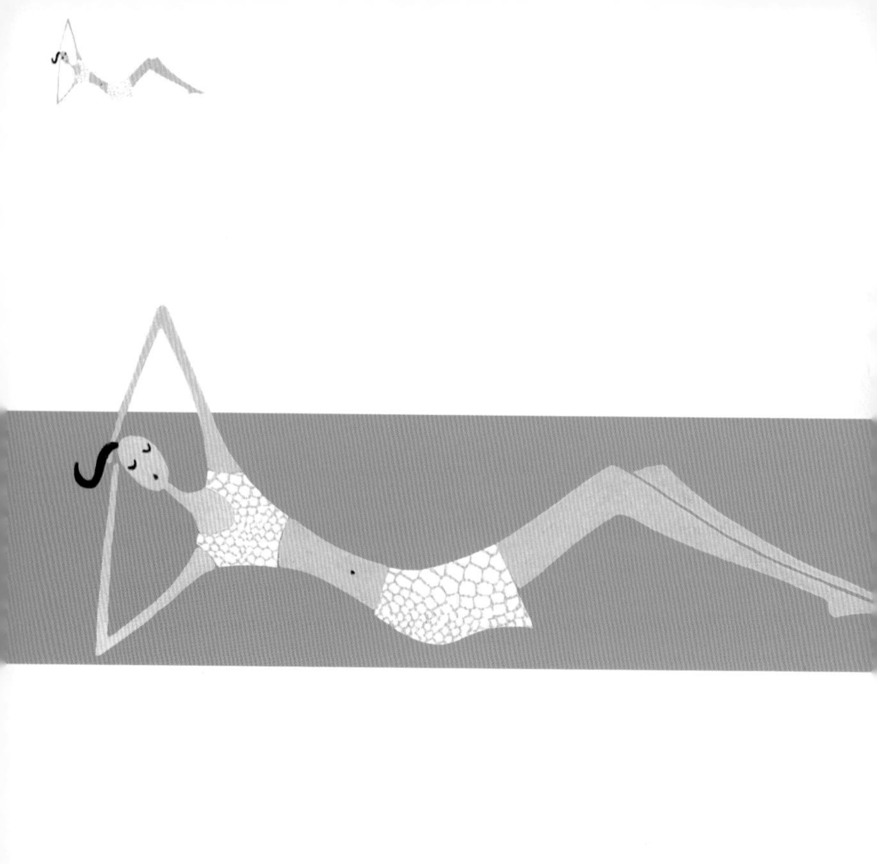

57 Tighten your stomach with these super-effective sit-ups:

1. Lie on the floor with your feet hip-width apart and hands by the side of your head. Without pulling on your head, breathe out and slowly lift your shoulders off the floor. Hold for a count of two, keeping your stomach tight, and then relax down. Aim for 15.

2. In the same position, raise your right leg and place the ankle over your opposite knee. Breathe out and slowly lift up, twisting your left elbow toward your right raised knee. Hold for two and lower. Repeat 10 times each side.

3. Lie on your back with your hands at the sides of your head, knees tucked into your chest and ankles crossed. Breathe out and slowly lift your shoulders while tucking up your bottom so your elbows meet your knees. Hold for two and relax. Repeat 10 times.

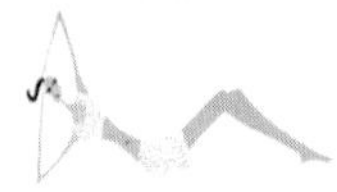

58 **Stretch your skin too far and the fibers will fracture.** The result? Stretch marks that zigzag across your stomach in thin, opaque white lines. These are most common during pregnancy or weight loss, so be prepared and massage in mandarin oil while your body's changing. This great-smelling oil can't guarantee to prevent stretch marks, but it makes a good moisturizer and it also speeds up cell regeneration. Mix 5 to 6 drops with 1 tablespoon of any vegetable oil.

59 **Bloating can make an otherwise trim tummy blow up like a balloon.** If you're a regular sufferer, chances are your diet needs changing. Try to eat regular meals, and don't eat on the run. Eating quickly or while talking is another factor; you gulp extra air as you swallow. Avoid fizzy drinks: All those bubbles will make you bulge. Other foods to watch out for are beans, cabbage, onions, and brussel sprouts. Any food can cause an intolerance—if you bloat up regularly, keep a diet diary for a week to see what's the problem.

60 **A swollen stomach just before your period** is due to water retention, and it's common to gain a few pounds in weight. Cut down on coffee, tea, and alcohol at this time and you should feel (and look) much better.

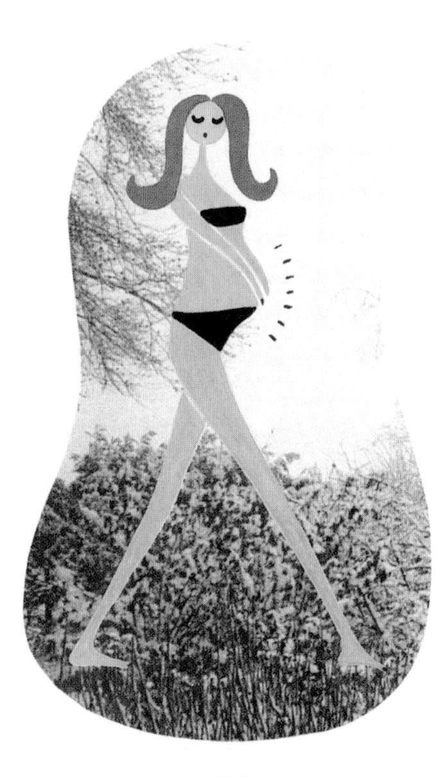

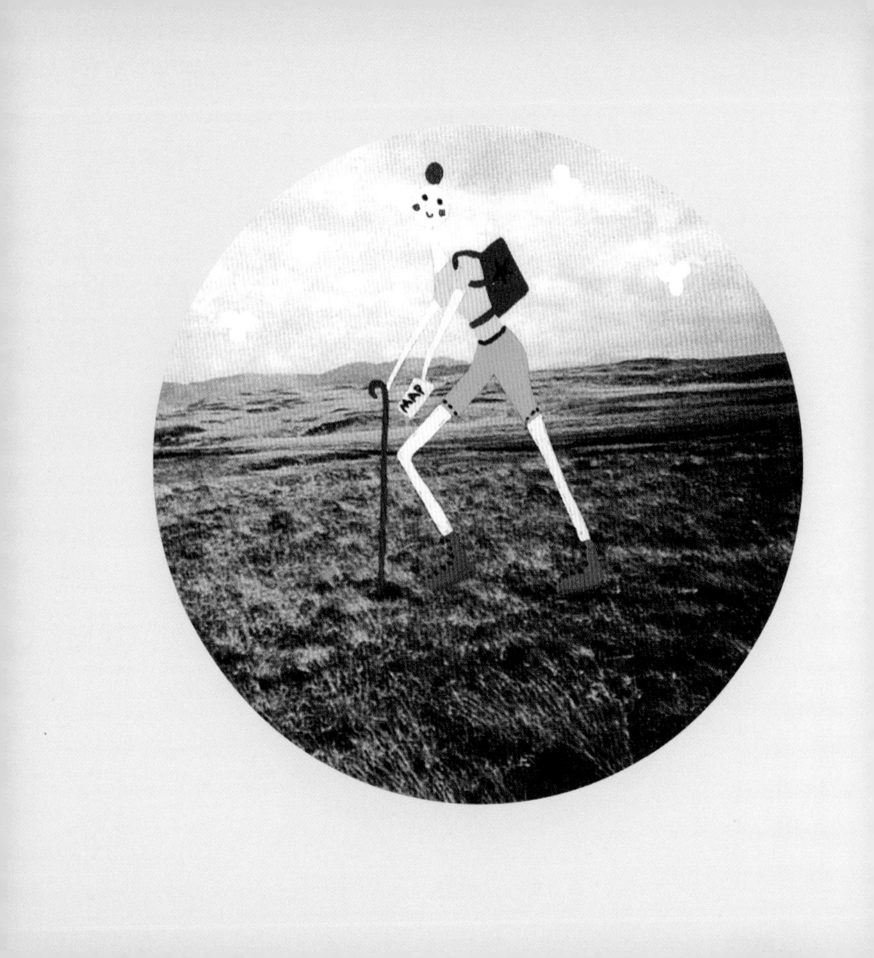
MAP

chapter 4

Lower body

61 **It doesn't matter how thin you are,** you can still have cellulite. Even skinny models can get lumpy, bumpy bottoms and orange-peel thighs. Cellulite can be caused by different things, and these can change depending on who you ask. But you can be sure that a bad diet, poor circulation, lack of exercise, and fluid retention won't help. The female hormone estrogen is also blamed for storing fat around the thighs, making them look dimpled. And the thinner your skin, the weaker the connective tissue that covers the stuff underneath. The result? A bit like a mesh shopping bag bulging with groceries. So how do you get rid of it? There are no easy answers here, but a combination of healthy eating, more exercise, and some massage should greatly improve matters.

62 **Anticellulite creams are big business.** They promise to make you into the model on the box. In reality you can only expect a cream to help strengthen the skin's surface, making the whole area look smoother. As for getting rid of the fat underneath, you're going to need to switch to a low-fat, high-fiber diet with plenty of water and fewer indulgences (such as sugar, salty, spicy foods, tea, coffee, and alcohol). No one said getting rid of cellulite was going to be fun!

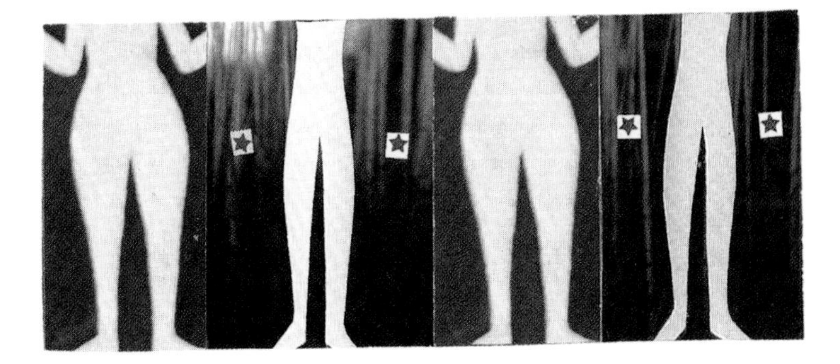

63 Water therapy (known as hydrotherapy in spas) can help smooth out a bumpy bottom. If you have a power shower spray, alternate bursts of cold water with warm, directed onto the problem areas. This speeds up the rate your body says goodbye to toxins and gives your circulation a kick start.

64 The right essential oil can help banish your body problems. Add one to your bath, or mix with a carrier oil for an all over massage.

- *Black pepper warms sore muscles.*
- *Cypress helps treat cellulite.*
- *Neroli promotes healthy circulation.*
- *Marjoram soothes stiff muscles.*
- *Mandarin eases fluid retention.*
- *Cedarwood treats aches and pains.*
- *Cinnamon boosts circulation.*
- *Grapefruit alleviates muscle fatigue.*
- *Lavender eases cramps.*

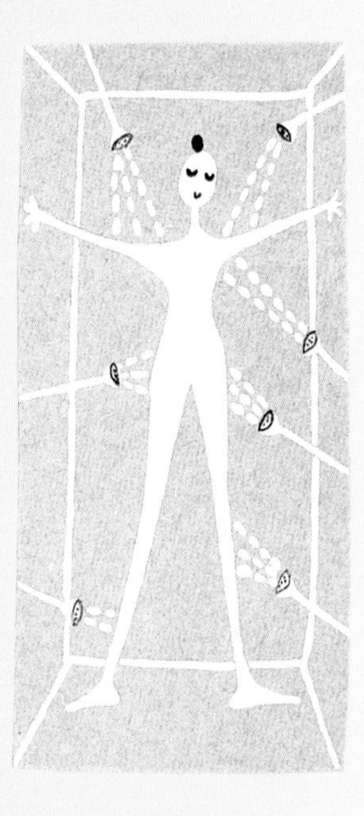

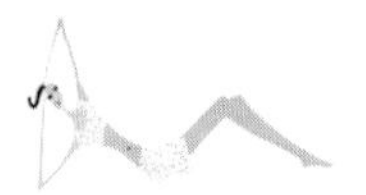

65 Copy this ballet move for toning hips and thighs:

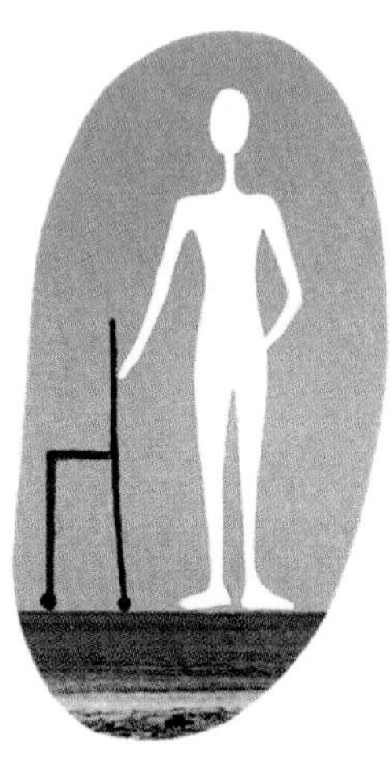

1. Stand up straight with heels together and hold onto a chair for support.

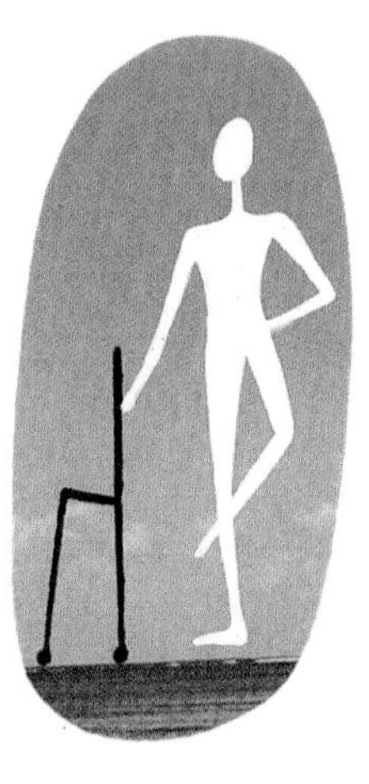

2. With your left leg slightly bent, lift your right knee up in front of you. Keep your body lifted and pull in your stomach.

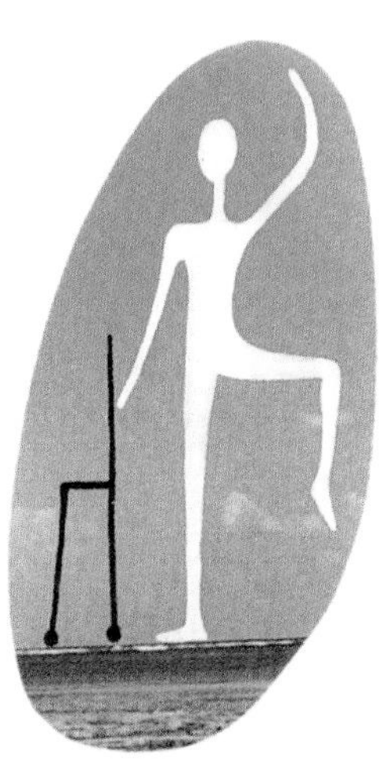

3. Bring your right knee out to the side, keeping your hips facing forward. For full ballet credentials, point your toe and lift your arm above your head, keeping the elbow slightly bent. Bring your leg down to the starting position and repeat 10 times on each side.

66 **Fed up with your pear-shaped body?** Well, at least it means you're healthier than apple-shaped people, who carry their weight around their middles. Pear-shaped people are less likely to suffer from heart disease, strokes, or diabetes, but make sure you keep your waist measurement less than half your height. There's nothing healthy about having a huge behind!

67 **Your bottom houses the biggest muscles of your body,** and the good news is they're very receptive to exercises like these:

Squats
Stand with feet shoulder-width apart and hands on hips. Keeping your back straight, extend your arms forward as you bend your knees and push your bottom out (imagine you're sitting on a chair). Slowly come up. Repeat 10 times.

Squeezes
Lie on your stomach with your knees bent and a ball between your feet. Turn your knees out to the sides slightly and squeeze the ball tightly. Open your knees a bit more and squeeze again. Keep going until you drop the ball.

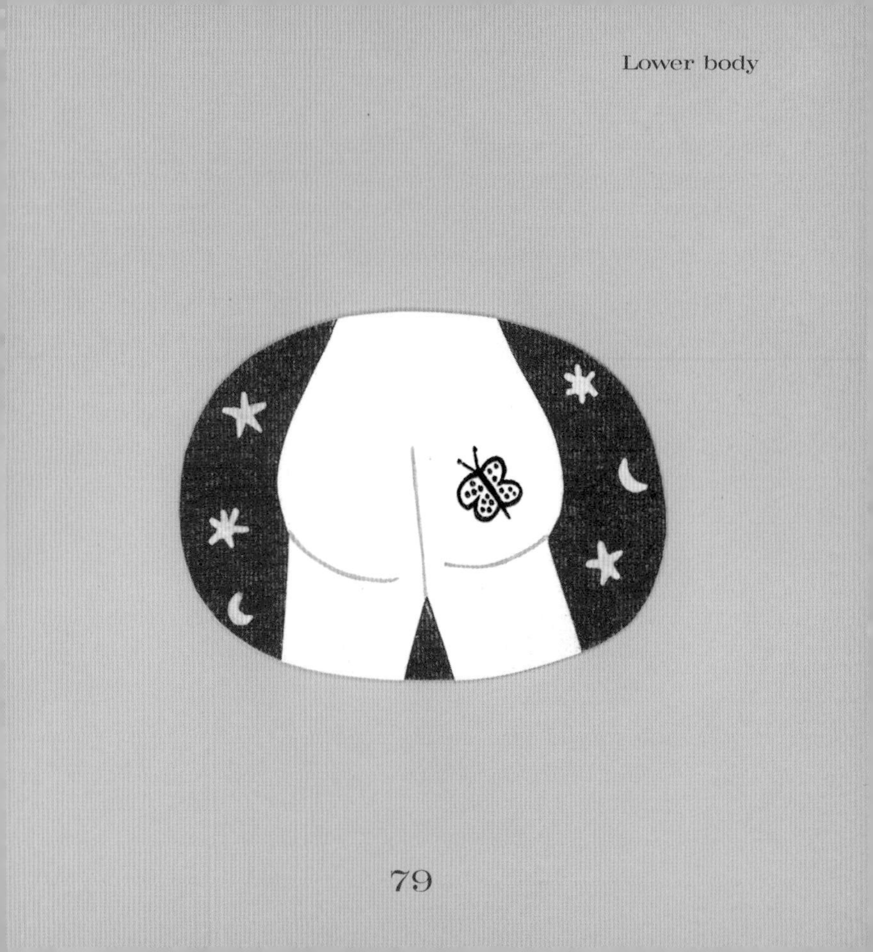

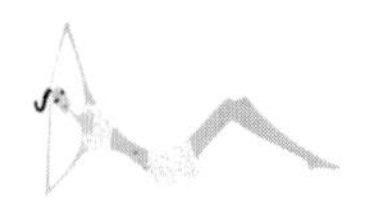

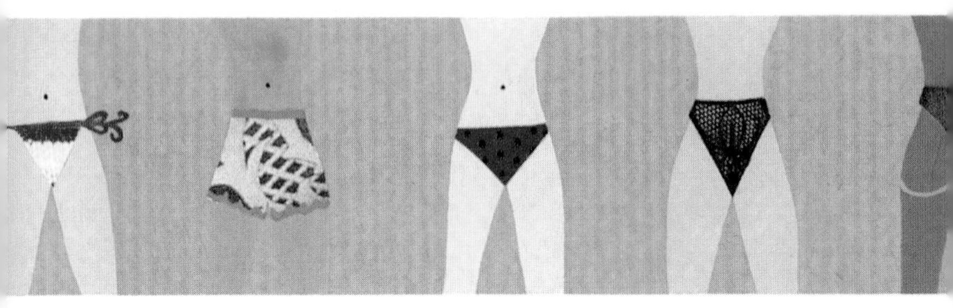

68 **To make the most of your bottom, wear the right panties.**

String bikini panties are two triangles with a string that connects over your hips. Avoid them if your hips are rounded since the string will cut your flesh in two and make you bulge out either side.

Control-top underwear holds your stomach in, but don't wear under anything too clingy. The excess has to go somewhere—you could be bulging out behind instead!

Bikini underwear has a waistband at hip level and suit everyone. Don't wear under clingy clothes as they will show through.

French-cut underwear is cut high on the legs, which has the advantage of streamlining your thighs and holding in your stomach. And when they're on show, they'll make your legs look longer too.

G-strings are the best panties to wear under clingy clothes, but they can feel uncomfortable at first. Try a few different styles—the width of the string is the crucial factor.

69 **For the ultimate invisible look,** wear pantyhose with a cotton crotch so you don't have to wear any underwear at all—just don't go out in a full skirt on a windy day!

70 Work off that flab with these simple leg exercises:

Step-outs
Stand with your hands on your hips. Take a step forward with your right foot and bend your left knee until it almost touches the floor. Repeat 5 times on each leg.

Leg-bends
Lie on your back with your legs in the air. Place the soles of your feet together and slowly bend and straighten your knees, keeping your feet together. Repeat 10 times.

Outer thigh lifts
Lie on your side with your legs straight and your hips facing forward. Lift your top leg as far as you can, being careful not to twist your hips back, then lower. Repeat 5 times on each leg.

Inner thigh lifts
Lie on one side with your bottom leg straight and your upper leg bent over the top so your foot's flat on the floor. Slowly lift your bottom leg up as far as you can, then lower. Repeat 5 times on each leg.

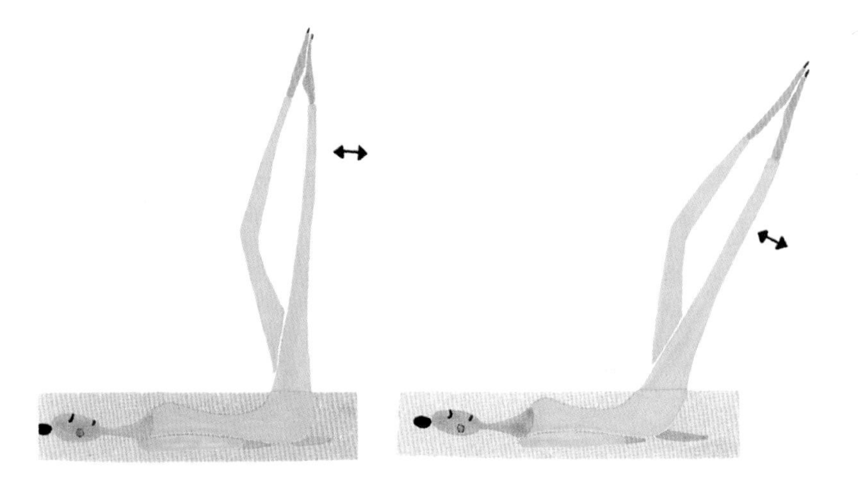

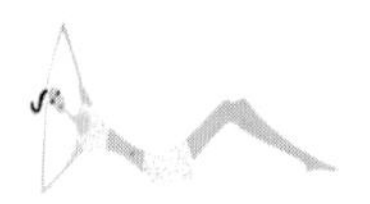

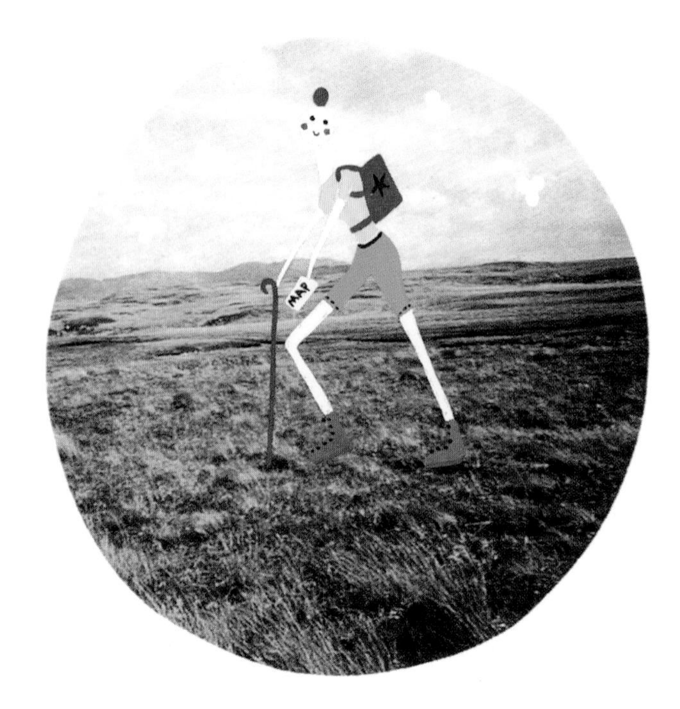
MAP

71 **Where a tight behind's concerned,** every little bit helps. Lengthen your stride as you walk so you're really moving along with arms swinging at your sides. Take the stairs rather than the elevator, or get off five floors early (as good as any step machine). And get on your bike for a brilliant butt work-out—set it on a low gear and pedal like crazy!

72 **Revive tired legs with a gentle shake at the end of a long day.** This will help get the blood pumping again.

73 **The skin on your legs has few oil glands, so it is the first area to dry up.** Combat crocodile skin with a rich moisturizer slathered on immediately after your bath or shower, while your skin's still damp.

74 **Do you regularly sit with your legs crossed?** Then you're doing your legs a massive injustice. Sitting with your legs crossed all day is a major contributor to blocked circulation, which can encourage spider veins and cellulite.

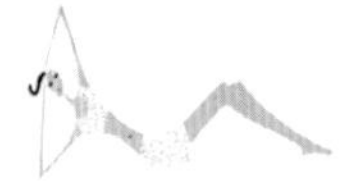

75 **White legs never look as long and slim as brown ones,** but don't be tempted to bake. The most common site for skin cancer on women is their legs. You have been warned.

76 **Around 20 percent of women suffer from varicose veins** (that's twice as many as men) thanks to pregnancy and weight gain. They can then be removed under local anesthesia through tiny incisions (ouch). Expensive, but you'll be pleased to know that once removed, the veins are gone forever (although you may develop more in time).

77 **When it comes to covering up less-than-perfect skin tone on your legs,** your average concealer just isn't up to the job. You need a professional cover cream that's waterproof and dense enough to hide everything from birthmarks to spider veins. Heavy-duty concealers can be found in all professional cosmetic stores, or ask your doctor for a prescription.

78 **The simplest exercise for a tighter butt?** Clench your buttocks and hold for five seconds. As long as you're not wearing anything clingy no one will be able to tell what you're doing!

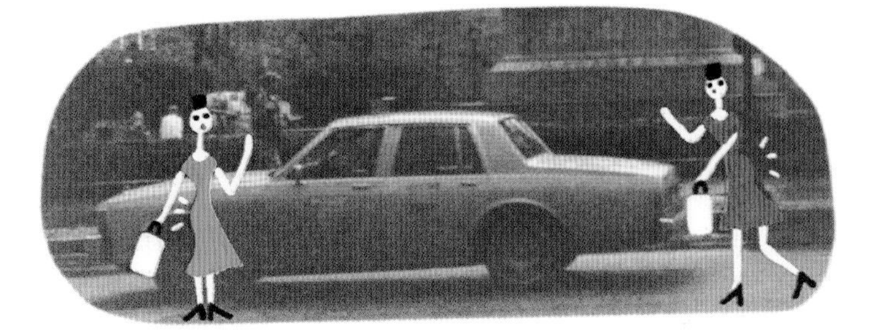

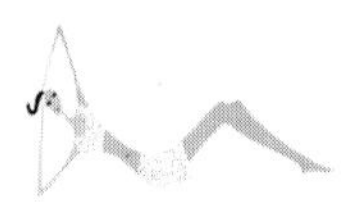

79 **If your calves are more straight than shapely**, try this easy exercise. Stand on the edge of a step with your heels hanging off the back, then lift up on your toes and slowly lower as far as you can go without toppling off. Repeat until you feel the burn.

80 **If you think your large lower half lets you down in photos,** try adopting the classic model's pose. Stand at a three-quarter angle—between profile and straight ahead. This will accentuate your good curves while hiding your bad.

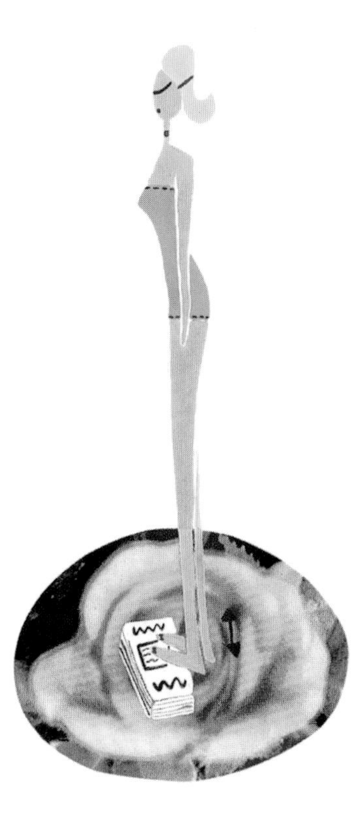

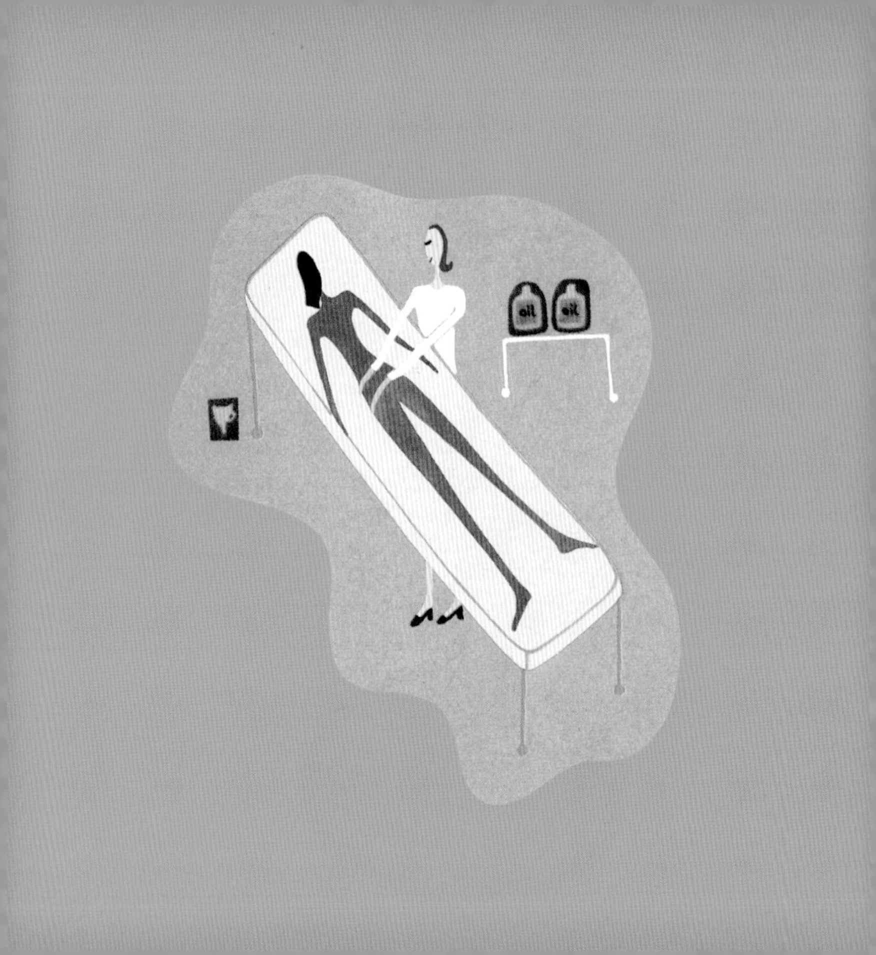
oil
oil

chapter 5

Body treats

81 **Ayurveda is the world's most ancient system of natural medicine** and is built on the balance of five cosmic elements known as *doshas:* earth, water, air, fire, and ether. Derived from these elements are the three *triodoshas: pitta,* which generates heat and governs the metabolism; *kapha,* which governs growth and structure; and *vata,* which generates all bodily movement. The health of the body is dependent on these three being in balance. An Ayurvedic expert will be able to tell you which of the *triodoshas* is dominant in your body and how to balance them accordingly. The purpose of Ayurvedic medicine is to promote health; many of its principles (eating fresh food and exercising every day) are now universally thought to prevent illness.

82 **Reiki is one of the fastest-growing therapies in the West** and promises to balance your body. To encourage relaxation and relieve aches, pains, and immunological problems, a practitioner places his or her hands on your body. Through the channeling of positive energy, painful areas can be soothed, and it's not unusual to feel deep warmth or tingling during treatment.

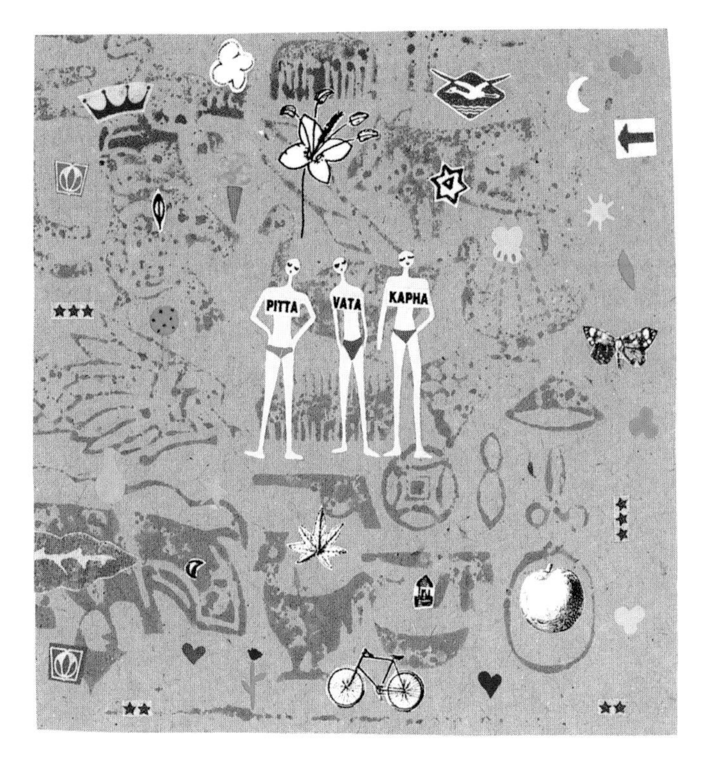
PITTA
VATA
KAPHA

83 **Hydrotherapy has been used for years to heal** and involves alternating temperatures of water varying from extreme cold to steam. The greater the difference in temperature, the more effective the treatment. Spas use underwater jets that start at the soles of the feet and work up the body to increase blood and lymph flow, which speeds up the rate at which toxins leave the body. A handheld jet is used for pummeling cellulite, to treat sports injuries, and to relieve aching muscles.

84 **For at-home healing for everything from stress to stretch marks, add essential oils to your bath.** Heat from the water dilates your capillaries so the oil is more quickly and easily absorbed. But be careful not to make the water too hot or the vapors will escape in the steam. Use no more than 6 drops total, and agitate the water well before stepping in because some oils (especially citrus) may sting the skin if not properly dispersed. Lie back and relax in the bathtub for 20 minutes.

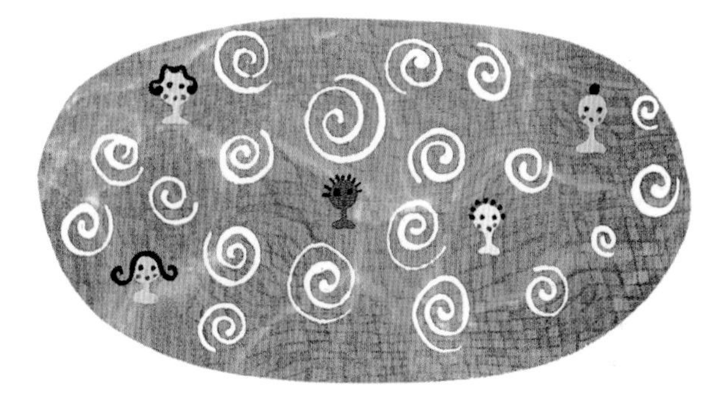

85 **Heat can be used to deep-clean and detox** by encouraging your body to sweat out toxins. Choose either a sauna (dry heat) or steam room (moist heat), and stay in no longer than 10 minutes. Avoid using this as a hangover cure: The heat will only dehydrate you more.

86 **To enhance your sauna experience,** add essential oils to the water that you pour over hot coals. Add 5 or 6 drops to 1 ladle of water, and don't sprinkle oil directly on the coals as it'll spit back at you. Choose pine essential oil to improve breathing and aid relaxation, cyprus or cedarwood to encourage detoxing, and antibacterial lavender or tea tree to fight infections.

87 **A hot, bubbling jacuzzi will help to ease aches and pains,** especially if you use a few drops of essential oil (don't use bubble bath; it will just foam like mad and clog up the jets). Try adding 4 to 5 drops of black pepper, cypress, lavender, or ginger essential oil to the water.

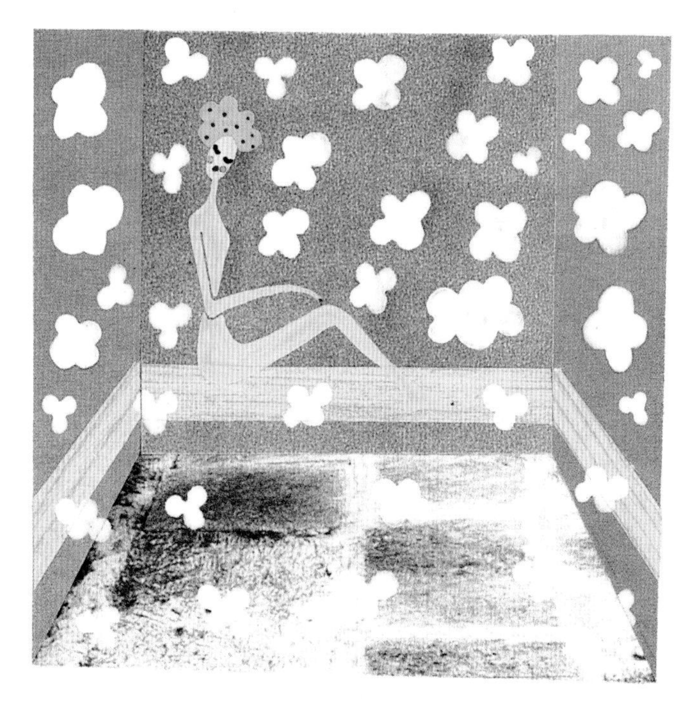

88 **Tanning ages your skin** and causes skin cancer, but it can make you look slimmer, hide minor blemishes, and even out skin tone. The answer? Fake it with a product that suits your natural skin tone (look for products labeled light, medium, or dark). Exfoliate and moisturize first to keep the cream from soaking into dry areas. Pay close attention as you apply the cream to remember where you've been—a double dose will leave you with streaks.

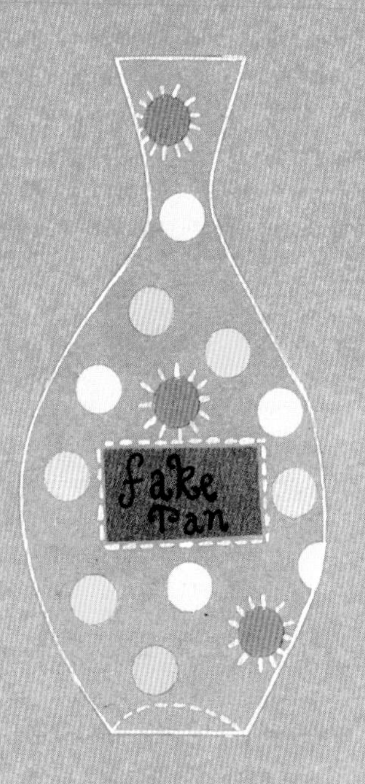
fake
Tan

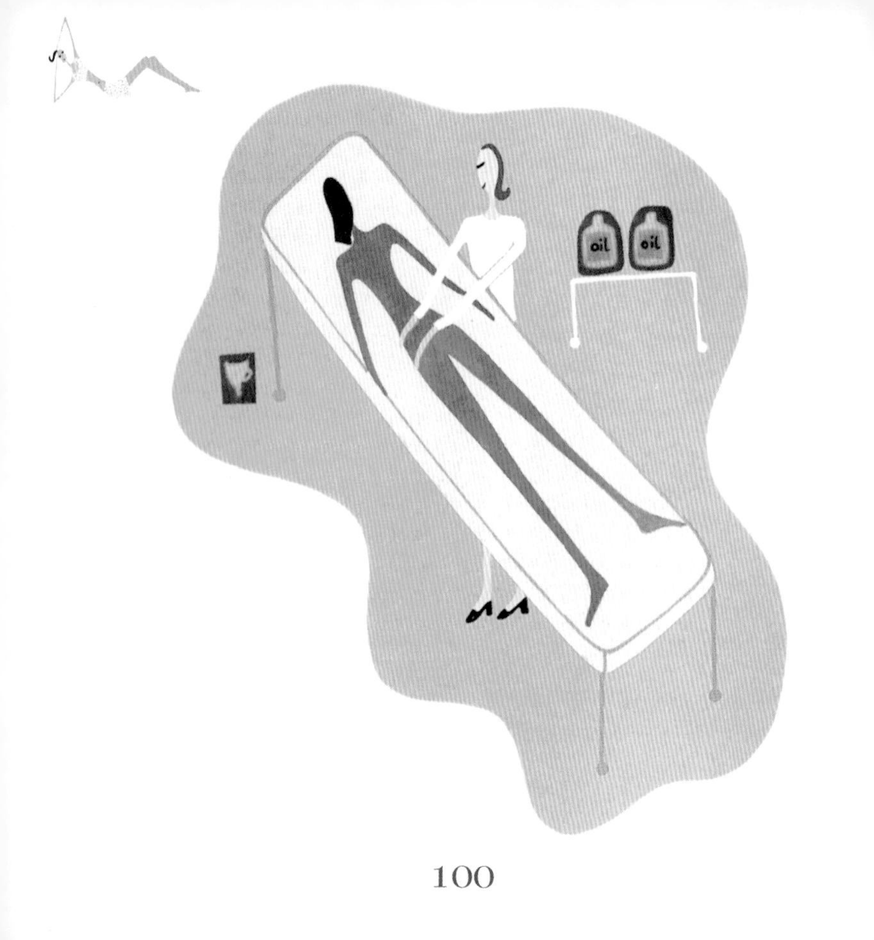
oil
oil

89 **The right massage technique can cure all kinds of ills.**

Thai massage concentrates on the pressure points to stimulate lymphatic drainage.

Swedish massage involves kneading and stroking the skin to relax muscles and stimulate circulation.

Reflexology treats the whole body by massaging reflex points in your feet to relieve health and emotional problems.

Holistic massage works on specific areas of your body related to different emotions to release stress stored in muscle and other tissue.

90 **Hands-on healing**—whatever your particular problem, there is a healing technique that will help to soothe it.

Cranio-sacral therapy is good for headaches, migraines and sinus problems.

Osteopathy helps tackle back and, joint pain, sports injuries, asthma, and PMS.

Chiropractic benefits those with spine and neck injuries, lower back pain, and painful periods.

Bowen technique is excellent for tension headaches and lower back injuries.

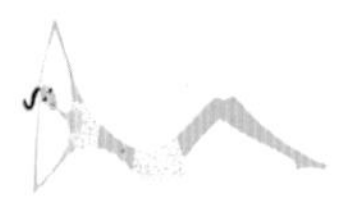

91 **A paraffin treatment will leave your skin supersoft and ease any aching muscles.** The warm wax is applied and your body is covered with a thermal blanket to generate heat and encourage the treatment to sink into your skin.

92 **Sesame oil is an anti-inflammatory and treats tired, over-worked muscles.** Massage a little in after a hard day when you need to keep going all night.

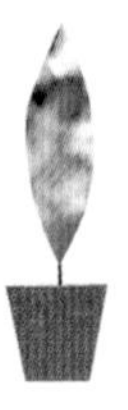

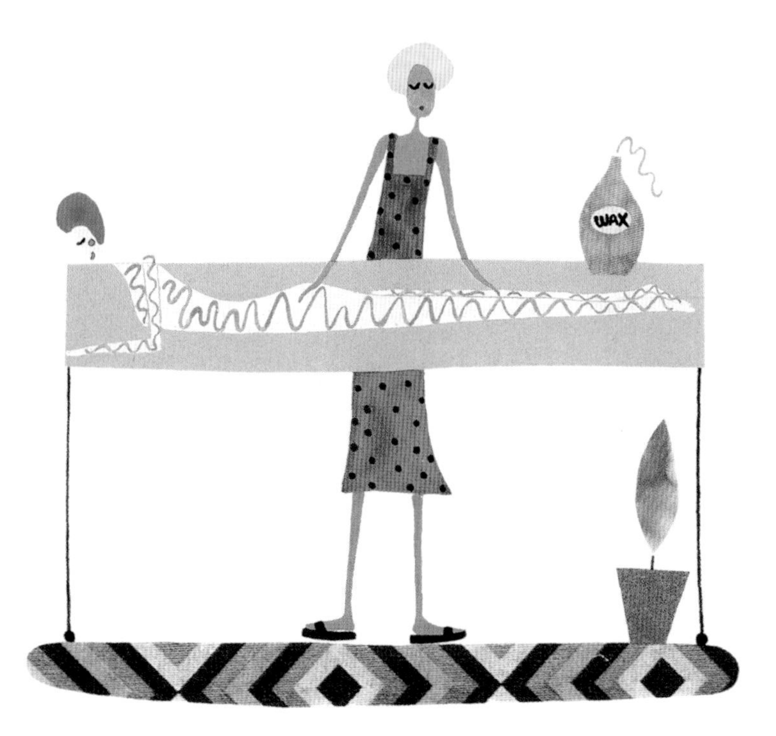
WAX

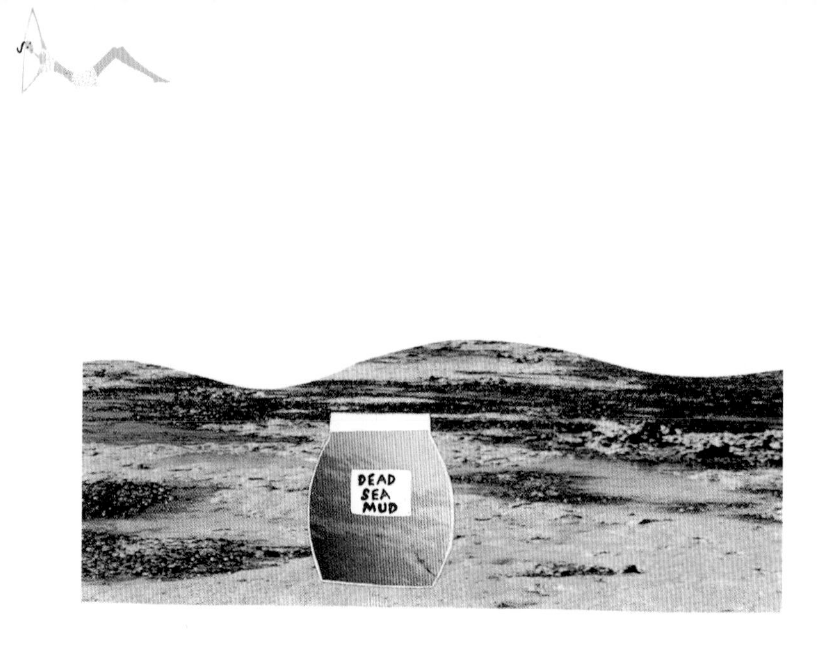
DEAD
SEA
MUD

93 **The kind of mud you find in beauty products has nothing in common with the stuff in your backyard.** These therapeutic muds are dug from deep in the ground and contain skin-friendly nutrients. The most popular mud is from the Dead Sea because it contains mineral salts 10 times more concentrated than in sea water. Medically proven to have healing properties, many European eczema and psoriasis sufferers make the Dead Sea their vacation destination every year. Mud is also a great detoxer and draws out all the dirt and grime. Make your own detox mud bath by mixing Fuller's Earth with warm water until it's muddy; lie in the water for 10 minutes.

94 **Make your own salt scrub to stimulate circulation** and deep-clean your body. Fill a cup with coarse sea salt and add water until you've got a thick paste. Then scoop up the paste with your hand and massage onto skin, avoiding delicate areas (think face, neck, and bust). Hop in the shower and rinse off, then wrap yourself in a towel and relax while those toxins pack their bags.

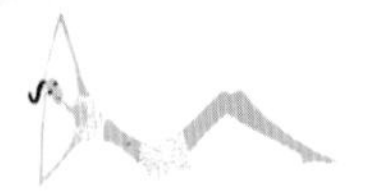

95 **Seaweed is a popular spa cure because it stimulates metabolism,** encourages fat burning, flushes out toxins, and boosts the immune system. You can buy seaweed bath soaks for an at-home detox treatment. Wrap yourself in a blanket afterward and rest for 10 to 15 minutes—you may feel a bit light-headed.

96 **One hour of flotation is said to provide the same deep relaxation as four hours of sleep.** And that's not all. Evidence has shown that lying suspended in a warm solution of Epsom salts greatly reduces blood pressure and heart rate, while lowering the levels of stress-related chemicals in your body.

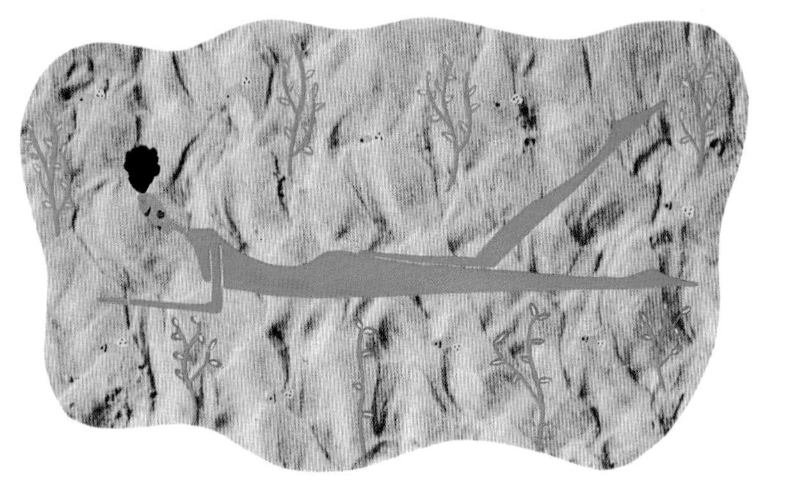

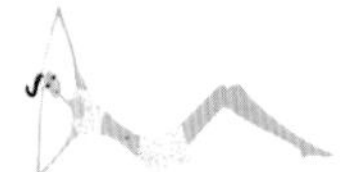

97 **The best way to start your day is with a freezing cold shower.** This will instantly wake you up and stimulate every part of your body, including your brain. Stay under for 30 to 60 seconds before turning the dial back to warm. Or do your own thermotherapy by alternating cold water with warm for 60 seconds each. Cold on the body sends blood to your organs and hot brings it rushing back to your muscles, which all adds up to a serious circulation boost.

98 **Treat your body to a fruit smoothie for breakfast**—nutrients are absorbed faster on an empty stomach. Blend together 1 banana, 1 cup of mineral water and 2 tablespoons of plain, low-fat yogurt and add whatever other fruit is available. Fruits that make a good smoothie include strawberries, peaches, pears, and oranges.

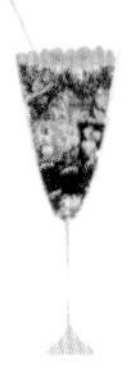

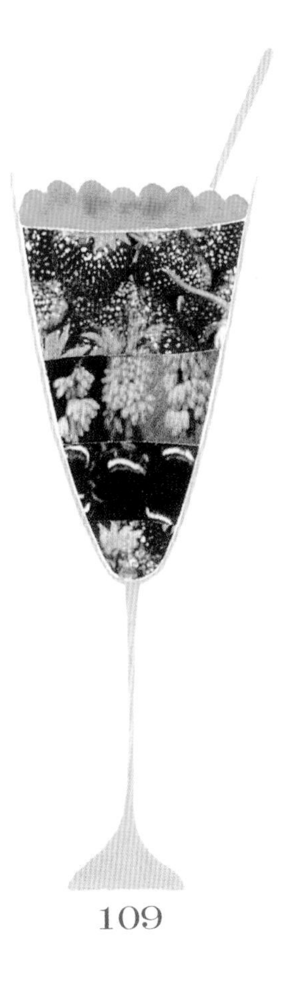

99 **Thalassotherapy is the word used to describe spa treatments using sea water** ("thalassa" is the Greek word for sea). Proponents say the minerals in sea water are similar to those in blood plasma, which means they are easily absorbed through the skin, especially when the water is heated to body temperature. Treatments include underwater massage, body wraps, and sea water baths, which increase energy, boost circulation, and tone your body by eliminating those pesky toxins.

100 **After all your hard work,** treat your body to a vacation (and show it off) or continue your good efforts and book a week at a spa for the ultimate getaway.

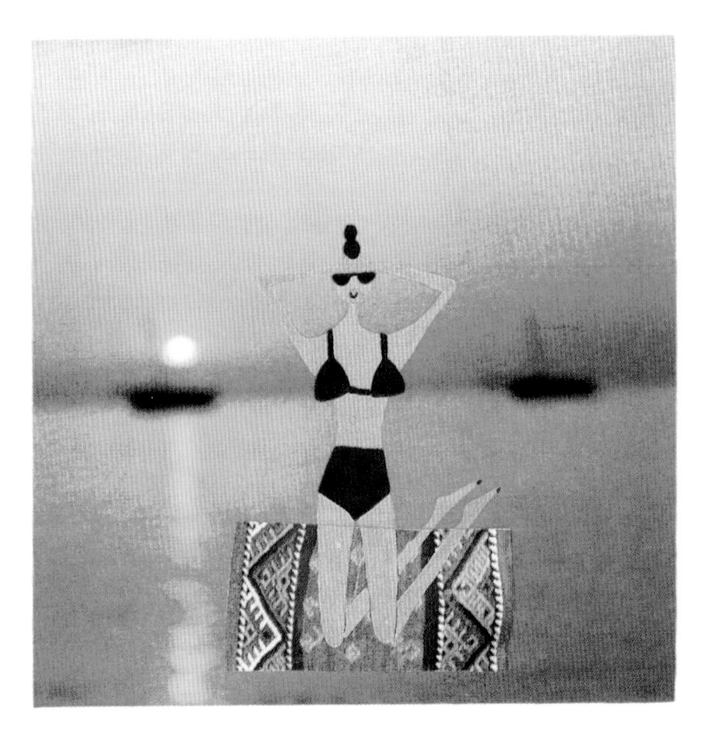

Cover design: Broadbase
Interior Design: The Big Idea
Series Editor: Elizabeth Carr

Time Warner Books are published by
Time Warner Trade Publishing
1271 Ave. of the Americas
New York, NY 10020

Visit our Web site at www.twbookmark.com

For information on Time Warner Trade Publishing's online publishing program, visit www.ipublish.com

 An AOL Time Warner Company

Printed in China
First printing: 10 9 8 7 6 5 4 3 2 1

Library of Congress Control Number: 2001094923

ISBN: 1-931722-02-1